T0212529

Communications
in Computer and Information Science   **632**

Commenced Publication in 2007
Founding and Former Series Editors:
Alfredo Cuzzocrea, Dominik Ślęzak, and Xiaokang Yang

Editorial Board

Simone Diniz Junqueira Barbosa
  Pontifical Catholic University of Rio de Janeiro (PUC-Rio),
  Rio de Janeiro, Brazil
Phoebe Chen
  La Trobe University, Melbourne, Australia
Xiaoyong Du
  Renmin University of China, Beijing, China
Joaquim Filipe
  Polytechnic Institute of Setúbal, Setúbal, Portugal
Orhun Kara
  TÜBİTAK BİLGEM and Middle East Technical University, Ankara, Turkey
Igor Kotenko
  St. Petersburg Institute for Informatics and Automation of the Russian
  Academy of Sciences, St. Petersburg, Russia
Ting Liu
  Harbin Institute of Technology (HIT), Harbin, China
Krishna M. Sivalingam
  Indian Institute of Technology Madras, Chennai, India
Takashi Washio
  Osaka University, Osaka, Japan

More information about this series at http://www.springer.com/series/7899

Jan Cabri · Pedro Pezarat Correia (Eds.)

Sports Science Research and Technology Support

Third International Congress, icSPORTS 2015
Lisbon, Portugal, November 15–17, 2015
Revised Selected Papers

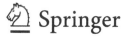 Springer

Editors
Jan Cabri
Norwegian School of Sport Sciences
Oslo
Norway

Pedro Pezarat Correia
Universidade de Lisboa
Cruz Quebrada
Portugal

ISSN 1865-0929   ISSN 1865-0937   (electronic)
Communications in Computer and Information Science
ISBN 978-3-319-52769-7   ISBN 978-3-319-52770-3   (eBook)
DOI 10.1007/978-3-319-52770-3

Library of Congress Control Number: 2017930146

© Springer International Publishing AG 2016
This work is subject to copyright. All rights are reserved by the Publisher, whether the whole or part of the material is concerned, specifically the rights of translation, reprinting, reuse of illustrations, recitation, broadcasting, reproduction on microfilms or in any other physical way, and transmission or information storage and retrieval, electronic adaptation, computer software, or by similar or dissimilar methodology now known or hereafter developed.
The use of general descriptive names, registered names, trademarks, service marks, etc. in this publication does not imply, even in the absence of a specific statement, that such names are exempt from the relevant protective laws and regulations and therefore free for general use.
The publisher, the authors and the editors are safe to assume that the advice and information in this book are believed to be true and accurate at the date of publication. Neither the publisher nor the authors or the editors give a warranty, express or implied, with respect to the material contained herein or for any errors or omissions that may have been made. The publisher remains neutral with regard to jurisdictional claims in published maps and institutional affiliations.

Printed on acid-free paper

This Springer imprint is published by Springer Nature
The registered company is Springer International Publishing AG
The registered company address is: Gewerbestrasse 11, 6330 Cham, Switzerland

Preface

This book includes extended and revised versions of a set of selected papers from the Third International Congress on Sport Sciences Research and Technology Support (icSPORTS 2015), held in Lisbon, Portugal, during November 15–17, 2015.

The purpose of the International Congress on Sport Sciences Research and Technology Support is to bring together researchers and practitioners in order to exchange ideas and developed synergies highlighting the benefits of any kind of technology for sports, either in general or regarding a particular case of application.

icSPORTS 2015 was sponsored by the Institute for Systems and Technologies of Information, Control and Communication (INSTICC). icSPORTS 2015 was co-organized by the University of Lisbon (Faculty of Human Kinetics), Portugal, and the Norwegian School of Sport Sciences, Norway, and had the institutional sponsorship of the Olympic Committee of Portugal. It was held in cooperation with the: European College of Sport Science (ECSS); European College of Sports and Exercise Physicians (ECOSEP); International Association of Computer Science in Sport (IACSS); European Federation of Sport Psychology (FEPSAC); European Society for Movement Analysis in Adults and Children (ESMAC); International Association of Sport Kinetics (IASK); European Society of Biomechanics (ESB); Portuguese Society of Physical Education (SPEF); European Association for Sport Management (EASM); Portuguese Sports Federation for Persons with Disabilities (FPDD); European Society for Sports Traumatology, Knee Surgery, and Arthroscopy (ESSKA); International Sports Engineering Association (ISEA); European Network of Sport Science, Education and Employment (ENSSEE); European Platform for Sport Innovation (EPSI.EU); Gait and Clinical Movement Analysis Society (GCMAS); International Society for Virtual Rehabilitation (ISVR); Portuguese Society of Physiotherapists (APF) and Sports Physiotherapy Group (GIFD); and Portuguese Society of Sports Medicine (SPDM).

icSPORTS 2015 also had as R&D group partners the following projects: REPOPA (REsearch into POlicy to enhance Physical Activity), Wi-Shoe (a novel wireless, wearable shoe-based system for real time monitoring of energy expenditure and gait parameters for sport and medical applications), and Credits4Health.

The congress received 93 paper submissions from 32 countries in all continents. To evaluate each submission, a double-blind paper review was performed by the Program Committee. After a stringent selection process, 15% of the submissions were published and presented as full papers, i.e., completed works (30-minute oral presentation), which shows the intention of preserving a high-quality forum for the next editions of this congress.

The congress program included panels, special sessions, and three keynote lectures delivered by internationally distinguished speakers, namely: Dietmar Schmidtbleicher (Goethe University, Germany); Romain Meeusen, (Vrije Universiteit Brussel,

Belgium), and Christian Finnsgård (Centre for Sport and Technology, Chalmers University of Technology, Sweden).

We would like to thank all authors whose research and development efforts are recorded here for future generations.

September 2016   Jan Cabri
                                                                       Pedro Pezarat Correia

Organization

Conference Chair

Jan Cabri   Norwegian School of Sport Sciences, Norway

Program Chair

Pedro Pezarat Correia   Universidade de Lisboa, Portugal

Program Committee

Duarte Araújo	Universidade Técnica de Lisboa, Portugal
Arnold Baca	University of Vienna, Austria
Abdülkerim Kasim Baltaci	Selçuk University, Turkey
José Angelo Barela	Universidade Cruzeiro do Sul, Brazil
Rodrigo Rico Bini	Universidade Federal do Rio Grande do Sul, Brazil
Daniel Boullosa	Universidade Católica de Brasília, Brazil
Jan Cabri	Norwegian School of Sport Sciences, Norway
Nick Caplan	Northumbria University, UK
Laura Capranica	Università degli Studi di Roma Foro Italico, Italy
Maria António Castro	Health School of Coimbra, IPC, Portugal
John Challis	The Pennsylvania State University, USA
Manuel Coelho-e-Silva	University of Coimbra, Portugal
Floren Colloud	Université de Poitiers, France
Rita Cordovil	Universidade Técnica de Lisboa, Portugal
Pedro Pezarat Correia	Universidade de Lisboa, Portugal
Nelson Cortes	George Mason University, USA
Giuseppe D'Antona	University of Pavia, Italy
Fernando Diefenthaeler	Universidade Federal de Santa Catarina, Brazil
Hayri Ertan	Anadolu University, Turkey
Vasileios Exadaktylos	BioRICS, Belgium
Timothy Andrew Exell	University of Portsmouth, UK
José Aurélio Marques Faria	Universidade da Beira Interior, Portugal
Peter Federolf	University of Innsbruck, Institute of Sport Science, Austria
Isabel Fragoso	Universidade Técnica de Lisboa, Portugal
Ronaldo E.G.D. Gabriel	University of Trás-os-Montes and Alto Douro, Portugal
Terry R. Haggerty	University of New Brunswick, Canada
Walter Herzog	The University of Calgary, Canada
Nicola J. Hodges	University of British Columbia, Canada
Patria Hume	Auckland University of Technology, New Zealand

Daniel James	Griffith University, Australia
Henrique Jones	Clínica Ortopédica do Montijo, Portugal
Larry Katz	University of Calgary, Canada
Andrew Kilding	Auckland University of Technology, New Zealand
Mark King	Loughborough University, UK
Andrey Koptyug	Mid Sweden University, Sweden
Nicola Lai	Old Dominion University, USA
Anthony Leicht	James Cook University, Australia
Silvio Lorenzetti	Institute for Biomechanics, ETH Zurich, Switzerland
Nicola Maffiuletti	Schulthess Clinic, Switzerland
Sandra Matsudo	Universidad Mayor, Chile
Kane Middleton	La Trobe University, Australia
Amir Ali Mohagheghi	Brunel University, UK
Fabio Nakamura	Universidade Estadual de Londrina, Brazil
Antoine Nordez	University of Nantes, France
Raul A.N.S. Oliveira	Universidade de Lisboa, Portugal
Matthew Pain	Loughborough University, UK
Pedro Passos	Universidade de Lisboa, Portugal
Carl Payton	Manchester Metropolitan University, UK
José Miguel Dias Pereira	Escola Superior de Tecnologia de Setúbal, Portugal
Alessandro Pezzoli	Politecnico di Torino and Università di Torino, Italy
Fernando Ribeiro	Universidade de Aveiro, Portugal
David Rowlands	Griffith University, Australia
Luís Silva	Universidade Lusiada, Portugal
Christos Spitas	Delft University of Technology, The Netherlands
Kazumoto Tanaka	Kinki University, Japan
Rui Torres	North Polytechnic Institute of Health, Paredes, Portugal
Herbert Ugrinowitsch	Universidade Federal de Minas Gerais, Brazil
Kirsti Uusi-Rasi	UKK Institute for Health Promotion Research, Finland
Jos Vanrenterghem	LJMU, Liverpool, UK
Benedicte Vanwanseele	KU Leuven, Belgium
J. Paulo Vilas-Boas	FADEUP/LABIOMEP/COP, Portugal
Hans Weghorn	BW Cooperative State University Stuttgart, Germany

Invited Speakers

Dietmar Schmidtbleicher	Goethe University, Germany
Romain Meeusen	Vrije Universiteit Brussel, Belgium
Christian Finnsgård	Centre for Sport and Technology, Chalmers University of Technology, Sweden
Federico Winer	STATS LCC, USA

Contents

Invited Paper

How Sports Can Create New Knowledge at a Technical University that Claim not Doing Research in Sport Science?

Christian Finnsgård[1,2(✉)]

[1] Centre for Sports Technology, Department of Physics,
Chalmers University of Technology, Gothenburg, Sweden
`christian.finnsgard@chalmers.se`
[2] SSPA Sweden AB, Research, Gothenburg, Sweden

Abstract. The purpose of this paper is to describe how a technical university have endeavoured into sports. This short paper will provide examples of a different approach to research in sports combined with technology. Chalmers University of Technology in Gothenburg, Sweden has for the last few years become engaged into research using sports as an application area for applied research. The research efforts has utilised the way that sports are organised in Sweden, with the sports confederations and clubs providing the problem areas to base the research around. For the university several aspects have been key in the research efforts. Chalmers will not do research in sport science, but all researchers will stay in their respective area of expertise. This short paper will focus on how this approach strengthens our research in diverse areas such as the automotive industry (with examples from production logistics and crash safety) for the forest industry (composites and cellulose research) and astronomy. But they have now all been further developed by sports.

Keywords: Sports and technology · Technical university · Technology · Sports

1 Introduction

The study resulting with the current paper is a part of an initiative at Chalmers University of Technology. The Olympic motto, "Citius, Altius, Fortius" (Latin for "Faster, Higher, Stronger"), governs everyday life for many engineers, and for the last few years Chalmers has supported a project that focuses on the possibilities and challenges for research combined with engineering knowledge on the area of sports.

1.1 Sports?

Sports technology is a rapidly growing field worldwide. New developments in materials science, sensor and measurement technology, smart textiles, and computation and modelling are rapidly implemented and employed to develop, facilitate, and monitor training. Advanced technology is today an integrated part of elite sports and is helping

© Springer International Publishing AG 2016
J. Cabri and P. Pezarat Correia (Eds.): icSPORTS 2015, CCIS 632, pp. 3–9, 2016.
DOI: 10.1007/978-3-319-52770-3_1

athletes to push their limits. At the same time, sports technology is increasingly being utilised by the broader public.

More and more citizens are practicing sports due to the well-known relationship between exercise and health. This has lead to an increased demand for items such as physical monitoring devices and functional clothing in the consumer market.

Sports technology is an intersection of demands on materials, measurement technology, and physical modelling, generating rapid technological innovation.

This background provides possibilities both for start-up companies and existing companies that hope to expand their product portfolios. The market for sports technology increases steadily, largely dominated by clothing and equipment. For example, consumer purchases of sporting goods in the USA in 2014 amounted to 64 billion USD [1].

In a global comparison, Sweden is lagging behind in the sports technology sector. The share of the turnover associated with Sports technology is below EU-average and also small in comparison to neighbouring countries.

Thus, there is a huge potential for growth within this area, accentuating the need for focused research efforts and competent development to bring forward innovations.

There is currently also a rapidly growing interest in academic research on sports technology. One of the main drivers behind this is that the sports sector is characterised by early adaptation. The distance from idea and invention to implementation is short, and new materials or devices can rapidly be evaluated by users in the field. This is in contrast to other fields applying advanced technologies, such as aviation or pharmaceuticals, where strict regulations can result in long lead times for implementation.

Thus, the sports sector is an ideal arena for utilisation of academic research, combining challenging requirements and conditions with rapid implementation of knowledge and inventions.

1.2   Methodology

This paper is a simple description of a new initiative, with a structure following a keynote lecture given at the 2016 iCsports conference in Porto, Portugal.

1.3   The Structure of the Paper

The paper is composed as follows: Sect. 1 provides the background to the initiative. Section 2 governs sports technology at Chalmers, while Sect. 3 gives a few examples. Section 4 outlines future directions and Sect. 5 addresses the unexpected. Section 6 finalises the paper with concluding remarks.

2   Sports Technology at Chalmers University of Technology

2.1   Why? Who?

The Swedish word "Engagemang" translates into a combination of dedication, commitment, and involvement. That motivation, so to speak, resembles the reason for our engagement in Sports and for the present efforts to get our faculty, students, technicians, and administrators involved in high quality work related to applying our knowledge in technology on sports.

Our alumni are called "Chalmerister" and have provided us with a worldwide network that still identify themselves with their technical university, thereby providing us with world connections through the ages. The willingness to combine your love of sports, whilst reconnecting with your university has proven an important factor and a motivator for why doing this.

2.2   What?

The initial efforts of this project focused on a few sports within which Chalmers had committed faculty with both a background and connections. Efforts were emanated in three sports: swimming, sailing, and equine sports.

Our actions in these sports have evolved into the activities described below: workshops, education, dual careers, research projects, and outreach activities.

2.2.1   Workshops

The project's modus operandi has been quite simple: gather representatives from the sport and ask them about common problems. The main means to achieve this is by organising public workshops to gather representatives from a sport. We ask them in advance what they think are the main challenges within their sport. Provided with these topics, we address researchers from our faculty with the headlines and topics from the sport. The researchers then provide insight into these problems based on knowledge within their own fields.

These workshops are held on campus (usually in our biggest lecture halls) in the evening, allowing people to attend just after work. Refreshments are provided. Usual attendance is between 100 and 450 people, and the events have lasted between 2.5 and 4 h. The only other voluntary lecture for the public at Chalmers with this level of attendance is when the Nobel laureates talks.

By organising these events, university researchers are provided with researchable topics, master thesis proposals, consultancy work, new project partners, and new contacts outside academia and within the sports industry. Furthermore, we give an echo into the sport what we do and encourage them to contact us on all levels. Finally, we get into contact with those from our faculty that are dedicated to the sport in topic of the workshop – and these are the ones that in the future will generate new contributions in relation to that sport.

We do empathically recommend that other institutions pursue this approach.

2.2.2   Education

The university has developed an advanced level course in "Sports Technology", which is given yearly at the advanced level. A great number of bachelor thesis projects and master thesis projects have been completed. Currently in 2016 we have over 60 students engaged in bachelor or master thesis work alone.

However, the biggest challenge is integrating sports and sports examples into the usual technology courses. The power of examples in visualising difficult engineering problems is a very pedagogical tool that can be repeated over time to enhance student learning.

2.2.3   Dual Careers

The focus on sports as part of the Chalmers strategy can be seen by the appointment of Chalmers and Göteborg University (in unison) as National Sports University (RiU, Riksidrottsuniversitet) [2] in the fall of 2015. The aim of RiU is to strengthen Sweden's international competitiveness in the sports sector and to enable athletes to combine higher education and elite sports careers.

2.2.4   Research Projects

Chalmers faculty and students have engaged in a multitude of research projects. Many of them are multidisciplinary, making discoveries in technology and engineering simultaneously. A few examples are provided in Sect. 3.

Hosting academic conferences is also an area worth mentioning. For the last few years, Chalmers has hosted one major conference each year. In 2015, we organised a conference for 200 participants with the Swedish Sports Confederation, Elitidrottskonferensen 2015.

2.2.5   Outreach Activities

As an outreach activity, sports is very rewarding, especially since society as a whole tends to have a very good awareness of sports.

To connect to the public at big events such as the Volvo Ocean Race 2015 (exhibition and race amongst the teams using 8 different materials), the annual science fair in Göteborg, and the Eurohorse 2016 (building and construction of a high-tech equestrian hurdle, measuring the height above the bar that each hoarse will jump with laser beams, as all being examples of successful outreach activities).

It is also clear how sports technology is as an important hub for public outreach. It is swiftly becoming an arena for increasing awareness of research and innovation for groups not normally exposed to higher education and research in general, and higher education in technology in particular. Connecting to new societal groups is a priority for Chalmers, is the use of sports for societal integration. Sports can act as an enabler in this endeavour.

2.3   Resulting Competitive Advantages

A few competitive advantages of sports technology research have gradually come to light:

- Recruitment – students, researchers, staff
- Using Chalmers' competence in an area with great public interest
- Strengthen cooperation and collaboration between staff, faculty, students and various Chalmers organisations
- New interface for contacts, e.g., clubs, federations, and industry
- Extensive challenges in research and a short distance between research and users

3   Examples of Results

Detailed below are a few examples of recent research efforts.

3.1   Detection of Damage in Equine Hoofs

Utilizing one of the most common thermal property measurement methods, a new method to detect structural inhomogeneity in materials has been developed.

Sub-surface structural variations in horses' hooves can be monitored in a non-invasive manner by applying this method.

The project includes the development of a device for diagnosis and prognosis of problems in hooves (cracks, abscesses, and keratomas). A patent application for this device has been submitted, and spin-off company started.

3.2   Injury Prevention

The challenge of one project was the frequency of injury to the chest when horse riders suffer accidents.

The problem was to make models of the security vests, horses, and hooves to fit a manikin. The research was made possible by the use of world-leading crash safety research from the automotive industry.

3.3   Real Time Motion Sensor for Swimming

University students and researchers developed a prototype real-time motion sensor system for swimming, enabling wireless communication over a water/air interface. The challenge was in measuring a swimmer's hand and body movements in the water through the transmission of signals in different media (water/air).

3.4   Horse ECG

A collaboration effort between Chalmers, GU, the University of Borås, and veterinarians at the University of Sydney, Australia has aimed to develop a smart textile sensor to monitor the full ECG of horses [3]. Licensing of the technology is underway.

3.5   Heel and Trim of an Olympic Sailing Yacht

Other research worked to optimise the heel, trim, and crew positioning of a Laser (Olympic class dinghy) through computational fluid dynamics and full scale experiments. The team used a combination of advanced simulation tools and the unique ship testing facility at SSPA on Chalmers Campus. The study was presented at the iCSports-conference in 2014 (Best Paper award) [4] and in three master theses [5–7].

3.6   A Paper Boat

Another research team developed a new biocomposite (48% cellulose in a thermo-plast matrix) that is 10% lighter but with the same strength as a traditional glass-fibre composite. It was demonstrated in the hull of an Optimist dinghy (Fig. 1).

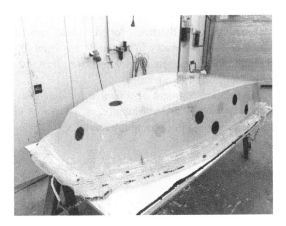

Fig. 1. An optimist built using a new bio-composite.

4   Starting in Three Sports and Moving on into Five Technology Platforms

As previously explained, Chalmers' sports technology research started in three different sports: swimming, sailing, and equine sports. Looking forward, we see five technology platforms, where we will combine our efforts in sports. These are:

- Lightweight composites in sports applications
- Sensors & big data
- Smart textiles
- Hydrodynamics in sports
- Injury prevention

Detailed descriptions of these lay outside the scope of this paper.

5   The Unexpected

This paper has described why, how, and what the Chalmers faculty should do to apply our knowledge in technology in sports. We anticipated that we would make contributions based on our knowledge in technology for the sports community. However, after only a few years of actions, and still claiming that we do NOT do research in Sport Science, an unexpected discovery has been made. As we apply our knowledge, researchers are now started using their experiences from this work to contribute back into our regular research within the university's ordinary fields of technology.

As with the few examples mentioned above, we now have a better grasp of motion analysis in production logistics, better development of crash safety manikins, and better research on mobile phone antennas.

Thus, research in sports has developed our knowledge in technology.

6　Concluding Remarks

We have endeavored on a journey for more and enhanced knowledge – not for sports, but for improving our knowledge about technology. Sports have proven over and over again to be an excellent means of doing this.

In this paper raises some cases of how simple solutions from sports pave the way for new technology. However, sports are not our beginning, and certainly not where we stop.

Acknowledgements. The author would like to express his gratitude to the financial support provided by Västra Götalandsregionen, Regionutvecklingsnämnden.

References

1. www.statista.com/statistics/200773/sporting-goods-consumer-purchases-in-the-us-since-2004
2. www.svenskidrott.se/Elitidrott/Riksidrottsuniversitet/, www.chalmers.se/sv/om-chalmers/samverkan-med-Goteborgs-universitet/Riksidrottsuniversitet/
3. McGreevy, P.D., Sundin, M., Karlsteen, M., Berglin, L., Ternström, J., Hawson, L., Richardsson, H., McLean, A.N.: J. Vet. Behav. **9**, 34 (2014)
4. Lindstrand Levin, R., Peter, J., och Finnsgård, C.: CFD prediction of the effect of appendages and leeway on the force trend of an Olympic class Laser dinghy hull. In: Cabri, J., Correia, P., Barreiros, J. (eds.) 2nd International Congress on Sport Sciences Research and Technology Support, icSports 2014, Rome, Italy, 24–26 October 2014 (2014)
5. Lindstrand Levin, R., Peters, J.: CFD Prediction of the Effect of Heel and Trim on an Olympic Dinghy (2014)
6. Pennanen, M.: CFD and VPP Optimisation of the Optimum Sailor Position on an Olympic Dinghy. Dept. Shipping and Marine Technology, Chalmers (2015)
7. Kostalas, K., Pluto, A.: Investigation of Sailing Yacht Forebodies in Head Seas. Dept. Shipping and Marine Technology, Chalmers (2015)

Papers

Gait Asymmetry During a 5-Km Time Trial in Elite Runners: A Descriptive Study

Rahel Ammann[1,2(✉)], Wolfgang Taube[2], and Thomas Wyss[1]

[1] Swiss Federal Institute of Sport Magglingen SFISM, Magglingen, Switzerland
{rahel.ammann, thomas.wyss}@baspo.admin.ch
[2] University of Fribourg, Department of Medicine,
Movement and Sport Science, Fribourg, Switzerland
wolfgang.taube@unifr.ch

Abstract. The present study evaluated gait asymmetry in elite runners by quantifying the differences between ground contact times (GCTs) of the right and left foot and its continuous changes over the course of a 5-km time trial on a 400-m synthetic track. By means of the inertial sensor Axiamote, the GCT of every step was assessed. The results revealed an overall gait asymmetry of 2.6%, but no changes in gait asymmetry over the course of the 5-km time trial. On the bend, the GCTs of the left foot were significantly ($p < .001$) longer than the GCTs of the right foot, whereas no such differences were reported on the straight section. However, gait asymmetry remained the same for both the straight and bend Sects. (2.7 vs. 2.8%). Overall, no gender differences regarding gait asymmetry occurred. In conclusion, a low and consistent gait asymmetry between GCTs of both feet in male and female runners was observed.

Keywords: Change over time · Bend versus straight · Inertial measurement unit · Field condition · Temporal progress of fatigue

1 Introduction

There are an impressive number of studies conducted on mechanics in running. Parameters of interest are among others step length, step frequency, breaking time, aerial time, and ground contact time [1–3]. Knowledge of these parameters is relevant for athletes, coaches, and researchers. The athlete and the coach need objective information to improve running technique and performance, whereas researchers need those running parameters to gain new knowledge about key performance indicators and injury risk factors. One possible risk factor identified in the literature is asymmetry of the lower limbs, which has been shown to have an impact on the incidence of injuries and possibly affect athletic performance [4]. However, the threshold at which a deficit becomes problematic remains to be defined. Some overall gait asymmetry might be normal, as the running style is automatized over the years of training and/or due to difference in leg lengths [5, 6]. In term of changes over the course of 5-km time trials, previous research showed significant decreases in stride length and frequency, while ground contact time (GCT) and total stride duration progressively lengthened [1, 7]. However, no former study investigated changes concerning gait asymmetry over the

© Springer International Publishing AG 2016
J. Cabri and P. Pezarat Correia (Eds.): icSPORTS 2015, CCIS 632, pp. 13–21, 2016.
DOI: 10.1007/978-3-319-52770-3_2

course of a maximal long-distance run. Such information might provide insight into the onset and progression of the athlete's fatigue and potential adaptations in running style. Gait asymmetry might not be evident during the start phase of a race, but might arise with the development of muscular fatigue. Furthermore, when running on a standardized 400-m synthetic track, the bend may be a potential reason for a certain overall gait asymmetry [8, 9]. In the scientific literature, bend running has received very little attention compared with straight track running, despite the bend portion being a considerable part of the whole running distance on an athletic track.

It is difficult to determine the most relevant biomechanical parameters to assess gait symmetry and asymmetry, respectively, as running depends on a variety of parameters. However, it seems reasonable to consider the ground contact time (GCT), as this is the only moment during running to generate propulsive force. The ability to produce and transmit high amounts of muscular force to the ground over a short period of time is a major determinant of the performance in running [10]. It was reported that runners with shorter GCTs were not only faster but also more energy efficient than runners with longer GCTs [3, 10, 11]. The less economical runners have lower vertical leg stiffness, which leads to enhanced braking time, and therefore, a longer GCT [12]. Hence, measuring GCT may be of potential benefit to investigate the presence of gait asymmetry. Previous research showed 3.5% gait asymmetry regarding GCTs in male Australian Rules football players, while running on a treadmill at their individual 80% VO2max [13]. Similar, Kong and de Heer [14] reported an average of 3.6% gait asymmetry between the GCTs of both feet in male Kenyan distance runners when measured at five different submaximal speeds on a treadmill. However, there is a lack of data that is obtained at maximal speeds during long-distance runs. This lack of knowledge should be counteracted as it was shown that with increasing intensity, step variability increases [15]. Moreover, all the aforementioned studies targeting gait asymmetry assessed GCT on the treadmill. It is well known that running on a treadmill changes running patterns [16]. Therefore, in order to make conclusions about functional relevant changes in gait asymmetry, measurements should be applicable in field conditions and during entire trials.

So far, no study has evaluated the gait asymmetry during maximal long-distance time trials on a 400-m synthetic track. Furthermore, the influence of fatigue on gait asymmetry in healthy female and male subjects is not known. The aims of the present study were threefold: Firstly, to quantify the gait asymmetry between GCTs of the right and left foot in elite female and male runners during a 5-km time trial on an outdoor synthetic track; Secondly, to examine the changes in gait asymmetry over the course of this 5-km time trial; Lastly, to evaluate the influence of running the bend versus running the straight track on gait asymmetry.

2 Methods

2.1 Subjects

A total of 10 female and 15 male (24.5 ± 3.4 years old, 174.8 ± 9.0 cm, 63.0 ± 8.1 kg) orienteers, competing at the international level, were recruited to participate in the study. All athletes were part of the Swiss Orienteering National Team and trained on average 14.1 ± 3.2 h per week. The local ethics committee approved the study and all participants provided written informed consent before testing. A medical questionnaire was administered to exclude athletes with any known lower limb injury in the past six months.

2.2 Procedure

The measurements took place during running a competitive 5-km time trial of the Swiss Orienteering Team. The time trial was one of the selection criteria for the participation in the upcoming world championships. After an individual warm-up session the runs were carried out on the 1st lane of a 400-m outdoor synthetic track with a radius of the curvature of 36.5-m [17]. The female and male runners started in two gender-segregated groups, and thereafter the gender groups were again split in half to avoid too many runners on the track at the same time. The athletes were free to choose their own pace in order to achieve the shortest time possible over the 5-km. Split times were provided every 200-m, including verbal encouragement. The time trials were performed in sunny weather, with no wind and air temperature constant at 24 °C. Running shoes were not predetermined; four athletes wore spikes and the other 21 wore minimal shoes. However, analyses for different shoe types were beyond the scope of this study.

2.3 Data Collection

Before testing, two Axiamote measurement units (Axiamo GmbH, Nidau, Switzerland) were attached, by means of customized elastics, to the shoe laces of the left and right foot of each subject. The Axiamote sensor (size: $3.8 \times 3.7 \times 0.8$ cm; weight: 13 g) consists of a 9-axis MotionTracking™ device MPU-9150 (InvenSense, Inc., San Jose, USA) that combines a 3-axial accelerometer, a 3-axis gyroscope, and a 3-axis magnetometer. Accelerometer data was recorded with a full-scale range of ± 16 g and a sampling rate of 1,000 Hz. Sensor operation and data transmission was established via Bluetooth, and data processing took place by the proprietary software. Good validity and reliability of the sensor in terms of GCT was recently demonstrated [18]. In order to assess split times per 200-m for every athlete, two video cameras (Handycam HDR-CX700VE, Sony Corporation, Tokyo, Japan) were placed alongside the track, one on the 200-m line and one on the finishing line.

2.4 Data Analysis

Running velocity and GCTs were averaged for each of the 25 segments of 200-m. Gait asymmetry between GCTs of both feet was computed as in Eq. 1 [19, 20].

$$\frac{|\text{GCT right} - \text{GCT left}|}{0.5 \cdot (\text{GCT right} + \text{GCT left})} \times 100 = \text{gait asymmetry } [\%] \qquad (1)$$

Only a subset of steps out of each 200-m segment was evaluated in order to differentiate between gait asymmetry on the bend and straight track sections. To ensure that GCTs from purely the bend and purely the straight track were included in the analyses of the respective section, the fifth to fourteenth step and the last fourteen to five steps of each foot per 200-m segment, respectively, were computed. Consequently, ten gait cycles each section were evaluated for running the bend and straight track section, respectively.

2.5 Statistical Analysis

Statistical analyses were performed by using SPSS Statistics 22 (Inc., Chicago, IL, USA) and the level of significance was set at $p \leq .05$. Data were expressed as overall means ± standard deviation and illustrated by means of boxplots. Gait asymmetry between GCTs of the left and right foot, straight and bend track section, and gender differences were calculated using paired and independent samples t-tests, respectively. The effect of running distance on gait asymmetry was evaluated by a repeated measures ANOVA on the 25 segments of 200-m and time*gender interactions. Furthermore, for comparison between straight and bend sections, also repeated measures ANOVA was applied.

3 Results

Mean 5-km performance time for both gender was 17 min 06 s ± 1 min 39 s (ranging from 14 min 43 s to 20 min 21 s), resulting in an average speed of 4.92 ± 0.48 ms^{-1} (Table 1). Men were running significantly ($p < .001$) faster than women and had significantly ($p < .001$) shorter GCTs. The measured gait asymmetry between GCTs of the left and right foot was 2.6 ± 2.1% without gender differences. Figure 1 illustrates the changes in gait asymmetry over the course of the 5-km time trial. The applied repeated measures ANOVA with a Greenhouse-Geisser correction revealed no significant changes over the 25 segments of 200-m ($F_{6,114} = 1.194$, $p = .317$) and no time*gender effects ($F_{6,114} = 2.194$, $p = .106$).

Table 1. Subjects' performance presented as means ± standard deviation.

	Overall	Women	Men
5-km time [min:ss]	17:06 ± 01:39	18:54 ± 00:56	15:55* ± 00:35
Speed [ms^{-1}]	4.92 ± 0.48	4.42 ± 0.26	5.24* ± 0.26
CV speed [%]	3.4 (1.9-6.1)	3.4 (1.9–5.0)	3.4 (1.9–6.1)
GCT [ms]	193.7 ± 14.3	199.3 ± 13.9	190.0* ± 13.3
Gait asymmetry [%]	2.57 ± 2.14	2.47 ± 1.79	2.65 ± 2.34

Note: CV = coefficient of variation in running speed per 200-m segment presented as mean (range); GCT = ground contact time; $^*p < .001$ between gender.

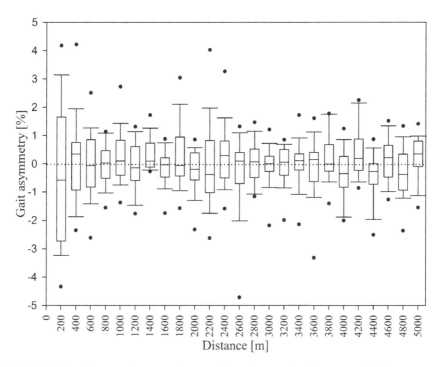

Fig. 1. Relative differences in ground contact times between both feet at each 200-m segment during the 5-km time trial. No significant gait asymmetry changes over the course occurred. For each boxplot the middle line represents the median value, the lower and upper limits represent the interquartile range, the error bars indicate the range and the dots denote the 5th and 95th percentiles.

Regarding differences in gait asymmetry between the straight and bend track section, GCTs on the bend were significantly longer compared to the GCTs on the straight track section (193.7 vs. 192.9 ms, $p < .001$; Table 2). Moreover, the GCTs of the left foot were significantly longer than the GCTs of the right foot on the bend (194.5 vs. 192.8, $p < .001$), whereas no difference in GCTs between both feet was shown on the straight section (193.0 vs. 192.9, $p = .876$). However, the relative gait asymmetry remained the same on the straight track section compared to the bend section with 2.7 and 2.8%, respectively. Repeated measures ANOVA did not reveal differences in gait asymmetry between the straight and bend track sections ($F_{1,291} = 8.602$, $p = .093$).

4   Discussion

The present study sought to examine gait asymmetry during running and its changes over a 5-km time trial. Furthermore, data were separately evaluated for straight and bend track sections of the 400-m synthetic track. Gait asymmetry was quantified by the

Table 2. Data on ground contact times (GCTs) of both feet separated by the straight and bend track section.

N = 625	GCTs both feet [ms]	GCTs left [ms]	GCTs right [ms]	Δ left-right [t-value; p-value]	Gait asymmetry [%]
Straight	192.9 ± 14.5	193.0 ± 15.3	192.9 ± 14.5	0.16; .876	2.7 ± 2.2
Bend	193.7 ± 14.5	194.5 ± 15.0	192.8 ± 14.7	6.10; .000	2.8 ± 2.3
Δ bend-straight [t-value; p-value]	3.81; .000	7.06; .000	−0.41; .680		0.238; .812

difference between the GCTs of the left and right foot. Overall, gait asymmetry in all elite orienteering athletes was 2.6%. This was less when compared to Brughelli et al. [13] and Kong and de Heer [14], who reported 3.5% and 3.6% asymmetry between GCTs of both feet, respectively. However, it is difficult to make direct comparisons between studies as the applied methodologies differed. The cited studies obtained data of male subjects on a treadmill at submaximal speeds. Moreover, subjects were Australian Rules football players demonstrating a different running style compared to athletic running specialists [13]. Lastly, data were measured during six step cycles only, which was reported to be very little, and therefore less reliable [14, 15]. The current 5-km time trial was executed under field conditions that automatically led to greater variability in pacing. This in turn might impact gait asymmetry even more. However, it appeared that the present elite athletes had smaller gait asymmetry despite running at maximal velocity over approximately 17 min.

Interestingly, the athletes in the present study kept gait asymmetry constant over the entire course of 5-km, because no 200-m segment could be detected as being particularly different from the others (Fig. 1). Related literature is lacking, as either gait asymmetry was not investigated or only over short sprint distances [1, 7, 21]. In previous research on sprint running it was recommended that data of distances longer than 30-m be obtained, because gait asymmetry might differ during different phases and/or at steady state running [21]. However, in the current study this assumption could not be confirmed, as no progression in gait asymmetry over time was observed. The elite athletes in the present study were able to consistently deal with the emerging fatigue and neither gender showed potential physical limitations by uneconomical and imbalanced behavior, which in turn could have increased injury risk or affected performance. Previously, it was stated that fatigue does not necessarily result in marked changes in kinematics during submaximal distance running [22]. Our findings support and extend this observation in that gait asymmetry was evaluated over the course of a maximal long-distance time trial. However, it has to be emphasized that the data were obtained in healthy runners. It might be assumed that athletes with previous or chronic injuries of the lower limbs are differently affected by fatigue and may show increases in gait asymmetry over the course of a race.

Throughout the time trial, the GCTs were significantly longer on the bend than on the straight track sections. More specifically, on the bend, the GCTs of the foot on the inside lane of the track (= left foot), were significantly longer than the GCTs of the right foot, whereas this difference did not exist on the straight section. However, the present study also highlights that the reported overall gait asymmetry cannot be explained by the bends of the circular 400-m track alone, because relative gait asymmetry remained the same on the straight compared to the bend track section with 2.7 and 2.8%, respectively. In previous studies investigating 200-m sprinting, asymmetries in kinematic movement patterns between left and right steps were larger on the bend than on the straight track [8, 9]. Moreover, Churchill et al. [8] demonstrated a decrease in sprinting performance on the bend due to reduced step frequency and increased GCT of the left step compared to the straight section. However, it was not known whether the bend had the same influence on gait asymmetry during sprinting and during long-distance running. Considering the significantly longer GCTs of the left than the right foot, the present results indicate that the bend has a similar influence on gait asymmetry during running at approximately 5 ms^{-1} as at 10 ms^{-1}, which was reported in the previous sprint study [8]. Nevertheless, in our study no mechanical explanations of force production can be provided, as the applied methodology was highly practical for field measurements in an entire group, yet, it has some limitations. Also, whether running performance differ between straight and bend track sections in long-distance runs needs to be examined in further research.

Individual gait asymmetry is masked when data is averaged for a whole sample, as in the present study. For example, depending on the athletes' individual running patterns, i.e., whether they tend to have a right or left foot imbalance, relative gait asymmetry decreases or increases when performing long-distance runs on an athletic track due to the bend. Furthermore, theoretically, some athletes could show higher gait asymmetry at the beginning and reduce this over the course of the race, while others may adapt in the other direction. Therefore, in high performance settings, data should be individualized so that personal strengths and weaknesses can be obtained for diagnostic and prognostic purposes. In case of gait asymmetry, targeted training interventions may be defined. In this respect, frequent measurements could be valuable, as classifying one's deficits after an injury is difficult when individual baseline data are lacking. For instance, having long-term data at hand would be useful for athletes, coaches, and medical staff to monitor rehabilitation progress or even to define a return to competition after rehabilitation.

The Axiamote sensor is a device with high practical application for enabling regular monitoring and evaluation of gait asymmetry in running. The small size and light weight allows data acquisition not only during training sessions but also during competitions. Additionally, data can be evaluated in real time even for a group of athletes.

5   Conclusions

The present study showed low and consistent asymmetry between GCTs of the left and right foot in healthy elite orienteers over a 5-km running time trial on a 400-m synthetic track. The athletes appeared to have the ability to deal with the emerging fatigue, as no alteration in gait asymmetry occurred over time. Furthermore, the GCTs of the left leg were significantly longer compared to the contacts of the right foot. Yet this alone does not explain the overall gait asymmetry, because relative gait asymmetry remained the same for both the bend and straight track section. Care should be taken when interpreting averaged data over a whole sample, and therefore, individual evaluation of gait asymmetry is recommended. The specified technology can obtain individual and long-term data to monitor gait asymmetry over single training sessions or entire training periods.

Acknowledgement. The authors thank the Swiss Orienteering National Team and the head coach Patrik Thoma for their effort, and the Swiss Athletics middle- and long-distance coach Louis Heyer for his expertise.

References

1. Girard, O., Millet, G.P., Slawinski, J., Racinais, S., Micallef, J.P.: Changes in running mechanics and spring-mass behaviour during a 5-km time trial. Int. J. Sports Med. **34**, 832–840 (2013)
2. Murphy, A.J., Lockie, R.G., Coutts, A.J.: Kinematic determinants of early acceleration in field sport athletes. J. Sports Sci. Med. **2**, 144–150 (2003)
3. Nummela, A.T., Keranen, T., Mikkelsson, L.O.: Factors related to top running speed and economy. Int. J. Sports Med. **28**, 655–661 (2007)
4. Croisier, J.L., Forthomme, B., Namurois, M.H., Vanderthommen, M., Crielaard, J.M.: Hamstring muscle strain recurrence and strength performance disorders. Am. J. Sports Med. **30**, 199–203 (2002)
5. Cavanagh, P.R., Williams, K.R.: The effect of stride length variation on oxygen uptake during distance running. Med. Sci. Sports Exerc. **14**, 30–35 (1982)
6. Gurney, B.: Leglength discrepancy. Gait Post **15**, 195–206 (2002)
7. Nummela, A.T., Heath, K.A., Paavolainen, L.M., Lambert, M.I., St. Clair Gibson, A., Rusko, H.K., Noakes, T.D.: Fatigue during a 5-km running time trial. Int. J. Sports Med. **29**, 738–745 (2008)
8. Churchill, S.M., Salo, A.I., Trewartha, G.: The effect of the bend on technique and performance during maximal effort sprinting. Sports Biomech. **14**, 106–121 (2015)
9. Alt, T., Heinrich, K., Funken, J., Potthast, W.: Lower extremity kinematics of athletics curve sprinting. J. Sports Sci. **33**, 552–560 (2015)
10. Weyand, P.G., Sternlight, D.B., Bellizzi, M.J., Wright, S.: Faster top running speeds are achieved with greater ground forces not more rapid leg movements. J. Appl. Physiol. **89**, 1991–1999 (2000)
11. Paavolainen, L., Nummela, A., Rusko, H., Hakkinen, K.: Explosive-strength training improves 5-km running time by improving running economy and muscle power. J. Appl. Physiol. **86**, 1527–1533 (1999)
12. Morin, J.B., Samozino, P., Zameziati, K., Belli, A.: A simple method for measuring stiffness during running. J. Appl. Biomech. **21**, 167–180 (2005)
13. Brughelli, M., Cronin, J., Mendiguchia, J., Kinsella, D., Nosaka, K.: Contralateral leg deficits in kinetic and kinematic variables during running in Australian rules football players with previous hamstring injuries. J. Strength Cond. Res. **24**, 2539–2544 (2010)
14. Kong, P.W., de Heer, H.: Anthropometric, gait and strength characteristics of Kenyan distance runners. J. Sports Sci. Med. **7**, 499–504 (2008)

15. Belli, A., Lacour, J.R., Komi, P.V., Candau, R., Denis, C.: Mechanical step variability during treadmill running. Eur. J. Appl. Physiol. Occup. Physiol. **70**, 510–517 (1995)
16. Nigg, B.M., de Boer, R.W., Fisher, V.: A kinematic comparison of overground and treadmill running. Med. Sci. Sports Exerc. **27**, 98–105 (1995)
17. Meinel, K.: Competition area. In: International Association of Athletics Federations, IAAF Track and Field Facilities Manual, pp. 31–54. Multiprint, Monaco (2008)
18. Ammann, R., Taube, W., Wyss, T.: Accuracy of PARTwear inertial sensor and Optojump optical measurement system for measuring ground contact time during running. J. Strength Cond. Res. **30**(7), 2057–2063 (2015)
19. Robinson, R.O., Herzog, W., Nigg, B.M.: Use of force platform variables to quantify the effects of chiropractic manipulation on gait symmetry. J. Manipulative Physiol. Ther. **10**, 172–176 (1987)
20. Zifchock, R.A., Davis, I., Hamill, J.: Kinetic asymmetry in female runners with and without retrospective tibial stress fractures. J. Biomech. **39**, 2792–2797 (2006)
21. Rumpf, M.C., Cronin, J.B., Mohamad, I.N., Mohamad, S., Oliver, J.L., Hughes, M.G.: Kinetic asymmetries during running in male youth. Phys. Ther. Sport **15**, 53–57 (2014)
22. Williams, K.R., Snow, R., Agruss, C.: Changes in distance running kinematics with fatigue. Int. J. Sport Biomech. **7**, 138–162 (1991)

Aerodynamical Resistance in Cycling on a Single Rider and on Two Drafting Riders: CFD Simulations, Validation and Comparison with Wind Tunnel Tests

Luca Oggiano$^{(\boxtimes)}$, Live Spurkland, Lars Sætran,
and Lars Morten Bardal

Department of Energy and Process Engineering,
Norwegian University of Science and Technology,
K. Hejes vei 2b, 7491 Trondheim, Norway
luca.oggiano@ntnu.no

Abstract. The present work intends to validate computational fluid dynamics (CFD) simulations to subsonic wind tunnel experiments. The models tested in the wind tunnel at NTNU (a mannequin and real cyclist in static position) were scanned using a 3D scanner consisting 48 single-lens reflex cameras surrounding the object in three heights (low/ground-midi-above). The simulations were obtained using the Unsteady Reynolds Averaged Navier-Stokes solver STARCCM+ from CD-Adapco. A hybrid meshing technique was used in order to discretize both surface and volume. Polyhedral cells were used on the model surface and in the near volume while a structured grid was used in the rest of the domain. An unsteady RANS approach was used and the turbulence was modeled using the Menter implementation of the k-ω model. The boundary layer was fully resolved and no wall functions were used and. The first part of the paper aims to validate the numerical model. In the second part CFD simulations were used to analyse the aerodynamic properties of two drafting cyclists varying the distance between them from 1 to 4 m with 1 m increments. A good overall agreement between the simulations and the experiments was found proving the value of CFD as a complementary tool to conventional wind tunnel testing.

Keywords: Aerodynamics · CFD · Wind tunnel testing · Cycling

1 Introduction

The aerodynamic drag is the main opposing force that cyclists need to overcome and it counts up 90% [1–3] of the total resisting forces experienced by a cyclist at racing speeds. The cyclist itself counts up to 70% of the total drag while the remaining 30% is due to the bicycle [3–6] and this leads to the fact that even small reductions could give large improvements in terms of performances.

The aerodynamic drag generated by the cyclist is directly linked to a number of parameters.

Expressing the drag as

© Springer International Publishing AG 2016
J. Cabri and P. Pezarat Correia (Eds.): icSPORTS 2015, CCIS 632, pp. 22–37, 2016.
DOI: 10.1007/978-3-319-52770-3_3

$$F_D = 0.5c_D\rho U^2 \tag{1}$$

It can be immediately noticed that, for a given location where the air density ρ [kg/m3] is assumed to be constant, the drag is proportional to the square of the wind speed U [m/s], to the frontal area A [m2] and to the non-dimensional drag coefficient C_D [-].

Being the frontal area measurements often not reliable [7], a combined parameter called drag area C_DA is used to quantify the effectiveness of a cycling posture.

In to order optimize their posture with the main goal to reduce the drag area (and thus the drag), experimental tests became common amongst elite cyclists. Different methods of assessment of aerodynamic drag (wind tunnel tests, linear regression analysis models, traction resistance measurement methods and deceleration methods) are currently used and each of them has pros and cons [7].

In addition to experimental methods, Computational Fluid Dynamics (CFD) simulations became a viable option due the increase in computational power available and to the possibility to parallelize the simulations splitting large meshes into smaller domains. Encouraging results from CFD simulations applied to cycling can be found in [4, 8–12] and while applications in other sports have been carried out by a number of other authors [13–15].

CFD simulations present some pros and some cons if compared with wind tunnel tests. While wind tunnel tests are able to provide only the total drag force acting on the model, CFD can provide drag information on individual body segments or bicycle components, increasing the insight in drag reduction mechanisms and allowing local modifications. Furthermore, CFD simulations are able to provide instantaneous field data while wind tunnel tests are not. On the other hand, the main disadvantage of CFD versus wind tunnel tests is that moving athletes are extremely complex to simulate and thus simulations are confined to static models. The other main issue is that, in order to reduce the computational cost of the simulations, turbulence has to be modeled and cannot be fully resolved. This simplification has two main drawbacks: the separation lines on the model will be placed considering the flow around the model fully turbulent (not always true in reality) and, even with the use of surface roughness and transition models, drag reduction techniques [16–20] cannot be simulated or directly implemented in the simulation.

The present work aims to validate CFD simulations towards experiments proving the effectiveness of CFD as a complementary rather than a substitute tool to wind tunnel tests.

2 Experimental Setup

Testing of the mannequin models and cyclist were conducted in the large wind tunnel at NTNU. The wind tunnel is equipped with a 220 KW fan engine, has a maximum speed of 30 m/s and the testing section is 2,7 × 1,8 × 12,5 m. A pitot tube and a thermocouple type K was used to monitor the wind speed and temperature respectively. The drag was measured with a Schenck six component force balance where only the axis of the drag direction was used. The drag force was calculated from the measured c_DA values and normalized.

2.1 Mannequin Model

The test on the mannequin model was conducted at five velocities ranging from 9.53 to 18.2 m/s (corresponding to 35 to 72,5 km/h).

The mannequin model used for the test was a full-scale upper body including head and upper arms belonging to a model of height 170 cm and weight 70 kg. Its position was adjusted to imitate that of a cyclist in the drop bars. The forearms were removed to reduce the amount of uncertainty and helmets were not included in the test. The model was tested with a number of jerseys with different surface pattern and without jersey with different rough patches applied to the shoulder.

2.2 Cyclist

The full-scale test on a cyclist was carried out at a single wind speed (13.09 m/s). A regular road bike was placed on a training roller so that the tires were not touching the wind tunnel floor and the roller was connected to the force plate. The front wheel was stationary and supported by a custom-made wheel stand. The cyclist was positioned in drop position with live pictures from a side camera projected in front of the rider showing the position superimposed with an outline of her initial position to keep it as consequent as possible.

3 Numerical Setup

3.1 Computational Domain and Geometry

The numerical simulations were set up for a cyclist without bicycle setup and for a mannequin without support setup. The bike modeling was discarded in order to reduce the mesh size and thus the computational cost of the simulation. However, due to this approach, the interaction between the bike and the cyclist was discarded and simplified. No roughness was added to the model while it has been previously shown that roughness could be a key factor and dramatically affect the drag [18–20]. The digital models for mannequin and cyclist were obtained using a high-resolution 3D laser scanning. The cyclist and mannequin digital models were placed in a numerical wind tunnel. A preliminary study on the domain size was carried out in order to avoid backflow that could affect the simulation. The domain shape and size is specified in Figs. 1, 2.

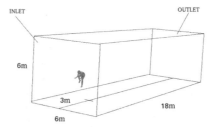

Fig. 1. Numerical wind tunnel.

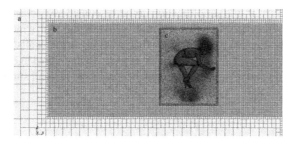

Fig. 2. Mesh refinement technique (a) far field area (structured mesh). (b) wake area (structured mesh). (c) Near model area (unstructured polyhedral mesh).

3.2 Mesh and Grid Sensitivity

A hybrid meshing approach was used to mesh the cyclist and the wind tunnel. A polyhedral meshing approach was used to discretize the models surface while a structured hexahedra approach was used for the rest of the domain. The polyhedral meshing technique allows smoother surfaces using fewer cells than triangular and tetrahedral meshing reducing computational cost. The boundary layer was resolved using an extruded mesh consisting of 10 layers. A growing ratio of 1.25 was used and the nearest cell to the surface was placed in order to ensure a non-dimensional distance from the wall $y+ < 5$, (where $y+$ is the distance y to the wall, non dimentionalized with the friction velocity $u\tau$ and kinematic viscosity v). This is needed in order to correctly resolve the viscous boundary layer in flows with high Re numbers. The models were contained in a near volume block of $L \times W \times H = 2 \times 2 \times 1.5$ m meshed with polyhedral meshing. A structured grid with a greed refinement in the wake area was used to model the rest of the domain. The near-model volume was patched with the rest of the domain using the overset mesh technique implemented in STARCCM+. The overlap region between the near model mesh and the domain mesh was chosen to me 10 cm. Three different surface meshes were used in a preliminary test in order to ensure a grid independent solution: a reference mesh consisting of 6.1 million cells approximately, a coarse grid consisting of 3.1 million approximately and a fine grid consisting of 12 million cells approximately.

3.3 Boundary Conditions

Standard boundary conditions suggested in the STARCCM+ guide were used for the current simulation [21]. A uniform flow inlet was used at the inlet. For the outlet, assuming the outlet pressure known and equal to the atmospheric pressure, and being the exact details of the flow distribution unknown a pressure outlet boundary condition was used. Symmetrical boundary conditions were used in sides, top and bottom of the domain assuming that on the two sides of the boundary, same physical processes exist. With symmetrical boundary condition, all the variables have same value and gradients at the same distance from the boundary and no flow across boundary and no scalar flux across boundary. Even if this simplification could be considered acceptable, one has to be aware that the numerical domain is simplified with the real wind tunnel. In particular, this assumption leads to the fact that friction at the walls, with the direct consequence of boundary layer growth, is neglected and blockage effects are not considered [22]. The model surface was modelled as a smooth wall surface with no slip conditions.

3.4   Solver Settings and Turbulence Modelling

The URANS turbulent flow solver implemented in STARCCM+ was used for the simulations and the k-ω Menter SST turbulence model was used for the simulations. A preliminary comparative study using the standard one equation Spalart Allmaras (SA) [23] and the two equations k-ω model [24] and the k-ω Menter SST [25] models was carried out and no noticeable differences between the use of the three models were found. Even if it is common knowledge that no single turbulence model can be considered superior for all classes of problems and thus the choice of turbulence model often depends on considerations such as the physics embedded in the problem, the level of accuracy required and the available computational resources, the choice was made based on comparisons carried out by other authors. The SA does not accurately compute fields that exhibit shear flow, separated flow, or decaying turbulence. Its advantage is that it is quite stable and shows good convergence. K-ω does not accurately compute flow fields with adverse pressure gradients, strong curvature to the flow, or jet flow. The k-ω Menter SST model does not use wall functions and tends to be most accurate when solving the flow near the wall. Furthermore, SST model also enables to capture the vortex structures developing in the wake region. For this reason, since large separation and vorticity is expected in the present test, the k-ω SST model was chosen [15, 26].

4   Validation Process (Results and Discussion)

4.1   Mannequin Models

The digital scanned model was positioned in the numerical wind tunnel in order to correctly reproduce the experiments position. The same simulation was carried out at six different wind speeds in order to correctly replicate the wind tunnel experiments and verify if the velocity could influence the drag area.

Validation against Experiments (Jersey on). The results show that CFD simulations consistently match experiments at different wind speeds with an error between simulations and experiments in the order of 10% which can considered to be a good agreement [4]. The results clearly show that the C_DA parameter is constant at different wind speeds allowing further simulations to limited to a single speed (Figs. 3, 4).

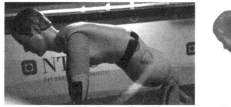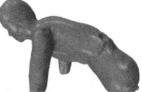

Fig. 3. Mannequin model in the wind tunnel (left) and 3D laser scanned model (right).

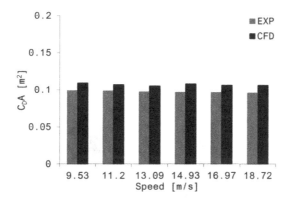

Fig. 4. C_DA values at different speeds for the mannequin with the jersey on for experiments (red) and simulations (black). (Color figure online)

Effect of Jersey on the Surface. Two different configurations of the model were simulated (with and without jersey) in order to evaluate how the jersey could influence the overall drag. The test was carried out at 14.93 m/s with the assumption that the drag coefficient would be constant at different wind speeds. Grooves and irregularities due to joints and mannequin construction were present on the model without jersey while these surface irregularities were either covered or smoothed in the scanned model with the jersey on (see Fig. 5). In particular bumps and imperfections on the back and shoulder area can be seen in the Fig. 5b while these imperfections are smoothed out in the model shown in Fig. 5a.

The measured drag from the mannequin without jersey resulted to be higher than the measured drag from the mannequin with jersey on (Figs. 6, 7).

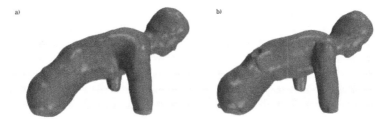

Fig. 5. 3D scanned model (a) model with jersey on. (b) model without jersey.

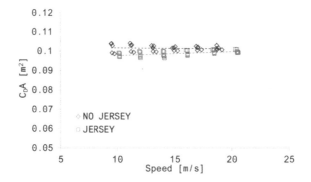

Fig. 6. Experimental results from the mannequin test with and without jersey.

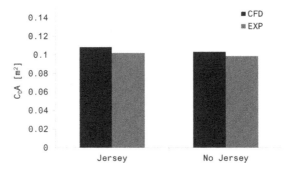

Fig. 7. C_DA values from experiments (red) and simulations (black) for the mannequin model with and without jersey at 14.93 m/s. (Color figure online)

The comparison between CFD and experiments presented in Fig. 8 shows the same trend seen in both experiments and computations with the main conclusion that placing a jersey on the model surface affects the flow around it and reduces the drag. The irregular surface on the plain model creates low-pressure zones that induce separation and recirculation of the flow with a consequent increase of pressure drag (Fig. 9). In particular, it can be seen in Fig. 8b that the wake area is larger than in Fig. 8a.

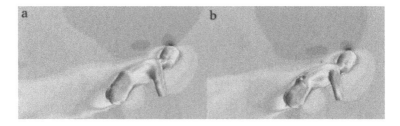

Fig. 8. Pressure contour plots on (a) the mannequin with jersey on and (b) mannequin without jersey.

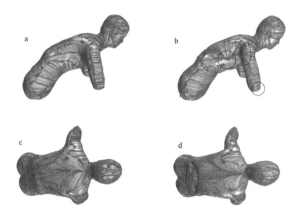

Fig. 9. Friciton lines on the model with jersey (a,c) and without jersey (b,d).

A high pressure area on the side of the model without jersey is also present while the same effect is not visible on the model with the jersey on.

The same findings can be seen when plotting the friction lines on the model. A recirculation area on the side of the model can be seen. This recirculation area is generated by the groove in the shoulder region where the arm is attached to the torso. From Fig. 10 it can also be seen that the flow on the arm separates differently on the model with jersey and on the model without jersey.

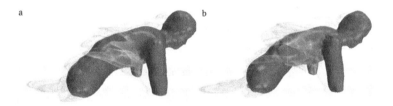

Fig. 10. Vorticity field around the mannequin model. (a) with jersey (b) without jersey.

Similar conclusions come also from where the vorticity field around the model is represented for visualization purposes. In the model with no jersey in Fig. 10b, the groove in the shoulder joint creates a vortex that develops and reattaches on the side of the model while the irregularities in the back induce separation.

4.2   Cyclist

Validation against Experiments (Dropped Position). Experiments were available only for the cyclist in dropped position. The drag of the bare athlete with no bike was obtained subtracting the drag measured for the bare bike from the drag measurements from the bicycle+cyclist test. While the experiments were carried out at three different wind speeds, a single CFD simulation at 13.09 m/s was carried out assuming the C_DA from CFD to be independent from the wind speed (Figs. 11, 12).

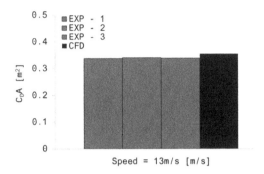

Fig. 11. C_DA values for the cyclist model from simulations (black) and experiments (red). (Color figure online)

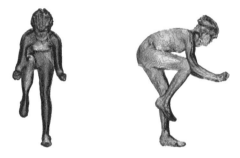

Fig. 12. Pressure contour plots on the rider.

The results from the CFD simulation match the experiments with an error of 10% and the simulated drag area C_DA is consistently higher than the measured one. The over prediction of the aerodynamic drag is a known problem in CFD simulations and it is directly linked to the turbulence modeling [4]. The standard turbulence models are in fact not able to correctly simulate the vortices in the recirculation regions and they often tend to keep the large structures without correctly resolving the smaller structures that are responsible of the vortex breaking mechanism, leading to an over prediction of the total drag.

Figure 13 illustrates the pressure field on the cyclist. The interaction between the different body parts can be seen in Fig. 14 where the vortices generated by the arms directly interact with the athlete trunk. Figure 13 also gives an overview of the area where separation might occur. The low pressure areas (blue color) are areas where the flow is detached. Large vortices are usually generated from these areas leading to an increase in total drag. Major attention to these areas is then important when designing a low drag suit.

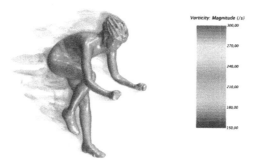

Fig. 13. Vorticity field around the rider. (Color figure online)

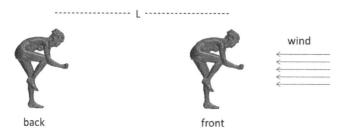

Fig. 14. Schematic representation of the two cyclists in tandem.

5   CFD Simulations on Two Drafting Cyclists

5.1   Description Setup

Once the numerical method was validated against wind tunnel experiments a parametric study with the scope of quantifying the total and relative drag of two cyclists positioned in tandem was carried out. The 3D scanned model used for the simulations was the model described in Sect. 4.2. The model was duplicated and translated a distance L Fig. 15. The simulations were run with the setup described in Sect. 3 and with distances L varying from 1 m to 4 m with 1 m increments. In the present study the bicycles were neglected. The total drag consisting of the sum of the pressure integration on the whole surface and friction drag was extracted for each distance L.

5.2   Results

The results from the parametric study show that it is beneficial to keep the distance L between the two cyclists as small as possible in order to reduce the overall drag. The back rider is located in a low-pressure zone due the velocity deficit caused by the wake

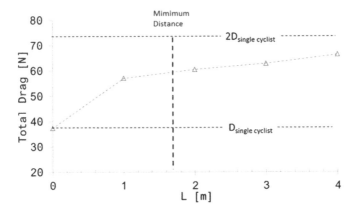

Fig. 15. Sum of the drag of front and back cyclist as function of L.

of the front rider. The low pressure behind the leading cyclist interacts with the area of overpressure in front of the trailing cyclist decreasing the under pressure area behind the leading cyclist.

The minimum distance achievable is however dependent on the bike size which by regulations cannot be smaller than 1.85 m. In principle, if the two riders could overlap each other, the total drag of the two riders would match the drag of a single rider. The drafting rider has the largest benefit from the tandem riding. On the other hand, if L is large, the velocity deficit would be small and the back rider would not benefit from his position.

While the lower drag experienced by the back rider can be clearly explained, the leading rider also experiences a drag reduction when riding in tandem. This was predicted and discussed by [4] and the results compare well with this study (Figs. 16, 17).

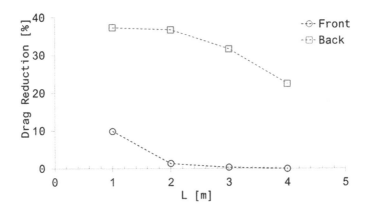

Fig. 16. Drag reduction for front and back rider as function of L.

Single Rider

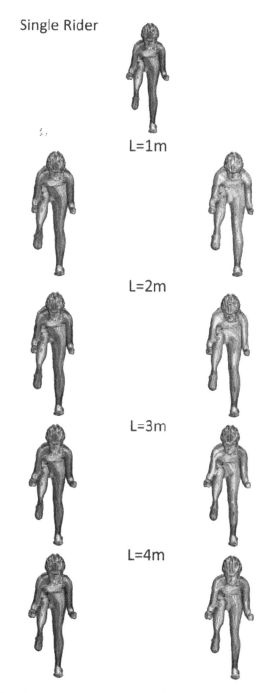

Fig. 17. Pressure plots on front (left) and back (right) rider.

A clearer picture of how the trailing rider is affected by riding in the wake of the leading rider is shown in Fig. 18 where the iso-pressure lines are plotted on both riders. While the differences in terms of pressure for the front riders are difficult to spot even of for the L = 1 m case, the differences in the second rider are more noticeable and it is clearly visible that the trailing rider experiences lower pressure and thus lower drag when L is small.

Similar conclusions can be grasped from Fig. 19 where the axial velocity field at the same time step is represented.

The drag reduction on the front rider is mostly due to an increase of pressure in the lower back area. This is a direct consequence of the fact that the two riders are so close that the front rider is located in the upstream low pressure area generated by the back rider. This increase in pressure can be seen in Fig. 18 where the contour plots for L = 1 m clearly show a large higher pressure area located in the lower back of the front rider.

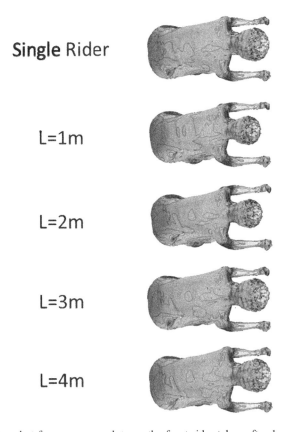

Single Rider

L=1m

L=2m

L=3m

L=4m

Fig. 18. Snapshot from pressure plots on the front rider taken after 1 s simulation.

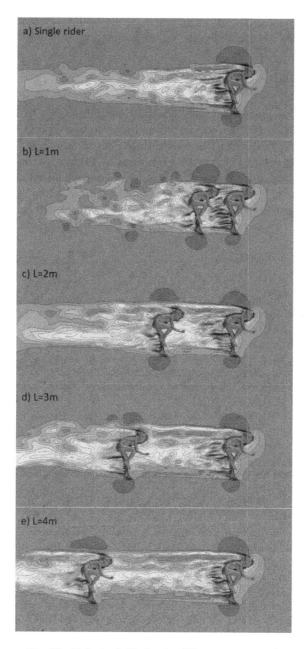

Fig. 19. Velocity fields for the different cases tested.

While for small distances L the trailing rider is in a low velocity (and consequently low pressure area), the velocity deficit is smaller for larger L leading to less reduction in drag. In Fig. 19b (L = 1 m) the influence of the trailing cyclist on the leading cyclist flow field can be seen. The disturbances from the trailing cyclist are propagated upstream generating a decrease in drag on the leading cyclist as well.

6 Conclusion

The simulated and experimental results consistently matched with an overall prediction estimated to be around 10% proving CFD simulations to be a useful tool. Wind tunnel tests are still needed for dynamic testing and surface modifications as CFD is restricted to static models and plain surfaces. On the other hand, CFD can give a greater insight to the pressure and force distributions on the model where wind tunnel experiments only provide the total drag force. CFD could therefore be used as a complementary tool to wind tunnel testing enhancing understanding of the flow patterns.

References

1. De Groot, G., Sargeant, A., Geysel, J.: Air friction and rolling resistance during cycling. Med. Sci. Sports Exerc. **27**, 1090–1095 (1995)
2. Di Prampero, P.E.: Cycling on earth, in space and on the moon. Eur. J. Appl. Physiol. **82**, 345–360 (2000)
3. Oggiano, L., et al.: Aerodynamic optimization and energy saving of cycling postures for international elite level cyclists. Eng. Sport **7**, 597–604 (2008)
4. Blocken, B., et al.: CFD simulations of the aerodynamic drag of two drafting cyclists. Comput. Fluids **71**, 435–445 (2013)
5. Underwood, L.: Aerodynamics of Track Cycling. The University of Canterbury, Christchurch (2012)
6. Underwood, L., Jermy, M.C.: Fabric testing for cycling skinsuits. In: 5th Asia-Pacific Congress on Sports Technology (APCST), Melbourne (2011)
7. Debraux, P., et al.: Aerodynamic drag in cycling: methods of assessment. Sports Biomech. **10**(3), 197–218 (2012)
8. Hanna, R.K.: Can CFD make a performance difference in sport? In: Haake, S.J. (ed.) The Engineering of Sport 4, pp. 17–30. Blackwell Science, Oxford (2002)
9. Defraeye, T., et al.: Aerodynamic study of different cyclist positions: CFD analysis and full-scale wind-tunnel tests. J. Biomech. **43**(7), 1262–1268 (2010)
10. Defraeye, T., et al.: Computational fluid dynamics analysis of cyclist aerodynamics: performance of different turbulence-modelling and boundary-layer modelling approaches. J. Biomech. **43**(12), 2281–2287 (2010)
11. Defraeye, T., et al.: Computational fluid dynamics analysis of drag and convective heat transfer of individual body segments for different cyclist positions. J. Biomech. **44**(9), 1695–1701 (2011)
12. Lukes, R.A., Chin, S.B., Haake, S.J.: The understanding and development of cycling aerodynamics. Sports Eng. **8**, 59–74 (2002)
13. Lecrivain, G., et al.: Using reverse engineering and computational fluid dynamics to investigate a lower arm amputee swimmer's performance. J. Biomech. **13**, 2855–2859 (2008)
14. Minetti, A.E., Machtsiras, G., Masters, J.C.: The optimum finger spacing in human swimming. J. Biomech. **42**, 2188–2190 (2009)

15. Zaïdi, H., et al.: Turbulence model choice for the calculation of drag forces when using the CFD method. J. Biomech. **10**(43), 405–411 (2010)
16. Oggiano, L., Sætran, L.: Experimental analysis on parameters affecting drag force on speed skaters. Sports Technol. **3**(4), 223–234 (2012)
17. Oggiano, L., et al.: Aerodynamic behaviour of single sport jersey fabrics with different roughness and cover factors. Sports Eng. **12**(1), 1–12 (2009)
18. Brownlie, L.: Aerodynamic characteristics of sports apparel, in School of Kinesiology. Simon Fraser University, Burnaby (1992)
19. Brownlie, L., et al.: Influence of apparel on aerodynamic drag in running. Ann. Physiol. Anthropol. **6**(3), 133–143 (1987)
20. Brownlie, L., et al.: Streamlining the time trial apparel of cyclists: the Nike Swift Spin project. Sports Technol. **1–2**, 53–60 (2009)
21. Cd-ADAPCO, STARCCM+ user guide (2015)
22. Chung, T.J.: Computational Fluid Dynamics. Cambridge University Press, Cambridge (2002)
23. Spalart, P.R.: Strategies for turbulence modelling and simulations. Int. J. Heat Fluid Flow **21** (3), 252–263 (2000)
24. Launder, B.E., Sharma, B.I.: Application of the energy dissipation model of turbulence to the calculation of flow near a spinning disc. Lett. Heat Mass Transf. **1**(2), 131–138 (1974)
25. Menter, F.R.: Two-equation eddy-viscosity turbulence models for engineering applications. AIAA J. **32**(8), 1598–1605 (1994)
26. Wilcox, D.C.: Turbulence Modelling for CFD, 3rd edn. DCW Industries, La Canada (2006)

Application of a Parallel Chain Platform to Provide Catching Practice in Cricket

Ajinkya Arun Bhole[1]([✉]) and Ravi Kant Mittal[2]

[1] Birla Institute of Technology and Science, Pilani, Rajasthan, India
ajinkya.b33@gmail.com
[2] K.R. Mangalam University, Gurgaon, India
rkm.krmu@gmail.com

Abstract. In the game of Cricket, there have been myriads of instances when dropped catches have resulted in lost matches. Catching requires great concentration, agility, hand-eye coordination and sure-handedness. Knowledge of good catching techniques alone does not suffice, ample practice is required to master the art of catching and building up confidence. Also, a rise in the number of unorthodox shots played by the batsmen in recent times has necessitated the requirement for a better and adaptable catching practice equipment.

This paper presents the application of robotics for providing a robust catching practice to the players. A redundantly actuated 2-DOF 3-UPS Parallel Chain Platform has been proposed for imparting catching practice drills to cricketers. This paper is an extension of the work presented by authors [1]. The basic idea is to swerve a ball shot from a Ball Shooting Machine onto the platform, in a random or pre-calculated direction by changing the orientation of the platform as the ball hits it. As compared to the presently available equipment, this equipment provides greater versatility and an increased degree of realism. We have formulated a methodology to provide practice drills for three types of catches, namely high catches, flat catches and reaction catches.

Keywords: Cricket · Training · Catching drills · Simulation and modelling · Parallel chain platform

1 Introduction

There are three main types of catches a fielder may encounter in Cricket: High catches, Flat catches and Reaction catches or catches taken close to the wicket. As with every other aspect of the game, sound technique gives the fielder an increased chance of success. Catching also requires a range of skills, some of which include intense concentration, ability to quickly react and excellent athleticism. Mastering these techniques and skills require intense practice of catching drills.

Application of technology to sports equipment has a great impact on performance and has a potential to revolutionize the entire sporting culture. To provide a better catching practice experience, we implement a 2 Degree of Freedom

© Springer International Publishing AG 2016
J. Cabri and P. Pezarat Correia (Eds.): icSPORTS 2015, CCIS 632, pp. 38–56, 2016.
DOI: 10.1007/978-3-319-52770-3_4

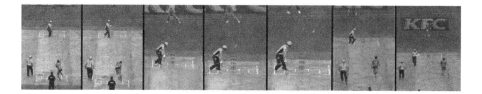

Fig. 1. The late-cut shot by Eoin Morgan.

(DOF) (Roll and Pitch) platform to direct a ball shot from a Ball Shooting Machine in random or pre-defined direction based on desired type of catch, ball speed, etc. This could pose an immediate question, why use a 2-DOF Platform separately along with the Ball Shooting Machine, as using a 2-DOF Ball Shooting Machine solely might serve the purpose? This can be answered if one looks at the unorthodox shot (Fig. 1) played by Eoin Morgan [4]. If one observes carefully, the wicket-keeper initially followed the ball by anticipating its trajectory, but did not keep an eye on the blade of the bat, and the brilliant late-cut shot by the batsman left him helpless. This is the reason why a wicketkeeper keep an eye on the ball as it the batsman's bat because they have a very small reaction time. Using a 2-DOF Platform for practicing catches creates an analogous situation as mentioned above. One of the keys to improving catching performance is to create a training exercise that holds a degree of realism, to accurately simulate what a player would face in the real performance environment. Here, the Ball Shooting Machine acts as the bowler and the Platform as the batsman's bat, thus, providing a degree of realism.

The paper has been organized into eight sections. Section 2 discusses the equipment and methods being used for catching drills and compares them with the proposed equipment. Section 3 provides a justification for picking a redundantly actuated platform for our application and also describes the details of the geometry of the platform and its Inverse Kinematic Analysis. Section 4 articulates details of our formulated method to calculate the velocity and angle of launch of the ball from the platform required for providing High Catches, Flat Catches and Reaction Catches. Section 5 discusses the nitty-gritties of the required velocity and angle of launch of ball shot from the Ball Shooting Machine. Section 6 discusses about the control input to the platform required to orient it for the desired catches. Finally, the simulation results are presented in Sect. 7 and conclusions and the scope for the future work are discussed in Sect. 8.

2   Current Catching Practice Methods

There are a number of methods and equipment in vogue to practice catching in Cricket. A traditional way of practicing catches is by shooting a ball on a pitch roller. The ball hits the curved surface of the roller and gets swerved for the fielder to catch, as shown in Fig. 2(a). This method is ineffective to provide a training for unorthodox shots as the fielder is able to predict the future trajectory of the

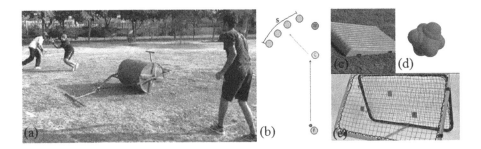

Fig. 2. Catching practice methods and equipment in vogue.

ball well in advance by observing where the ball lands on the curved surface. Another realistic way to practice slip catching requires a well-practiced coach to make it worthwhile. As shown in Fig. 2(b), the feeder (F) throws the ball such that it reaches the coach (C) at chest height, wide to the off side and the coach deflects the ball with a bat into the slip cordon (S) for practicing catches (Hinchliffe, 2010). A practice for high catches and flat catches can similarly be provided by an experienced coach. A Katchet, Reflex Ball and the Crazy Catch, shown in Fig. 2(c, d and e), are some devices that are used for practicing catches. These methods deflect the ball in unpredictable directions giving the fielder a good catching practice. But with these devices, it is very difficult to send the ball in desired directions, at desired angle or with desired velocity to practice specific type of catches. Sending the ball in desired manner is required to practice specifically on players weak spots.

These existing methods are heavily dependent on coach and do not provide any controlled training for practicing catches. Our proposed method does not depend on a coach, can provide catches in unpredictable as well as desired directions and with a degree of realism, thus providing a controlled and robust catching practice drills.

3 Design, Geometry and Inverse Kinematic Analysis of the Platform

3.1 Design

There are two choices for the architecture of 2-DOF platform, a Serial Chain or a Parallel Chain [3] as shown in Fig. 3, the End-Effector is the Platform. Parallel chain platforms have high payload capacity, are stiffer, faster, and more accurate than serial ones, and this architecture is suitable for current application. We have assumed that Ball Shooting Machine has a rotary degree of freedom and is able to shoot the ball accurately on the centre the platform. Hence, there is no requirement for translational degrees of freedom for the platform and the two rotational degrees of freedom i.e. roll and pitch are sufficient to direct the ball in desired directions.

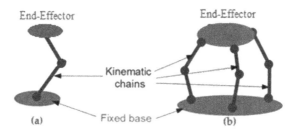

Fig. 3. Serial and parallel chain platforms (a) A serial chain platform (b) A parallel chain platform.

An obvious choice is, therefore, a 2-DOF Parallel Mechanism. Redundant actuation and novel redundant kinematics of parallel mechanisms are discussed by Andreas Muller [5]. Redundant actuation of the platform increases the payload and acceleration, and can yield an optimal load distribution among the actuators. It also promises to improve platform stiffness, dexterity and reliability. This led us to use and explore the 2-DOF redundantly actuated 3-UPS (Universal Joint–Prismatic Joint–Spherical Joint) parallel mechanism to manipulate the ball for catching practice. A CAD model of the proposed Redundantly Actuated 2-DOF 3-UPS Parallel Platform is shown in Fig. 4.

The design consists of a platform, a fixed base, three identical limbs, and a central strut connected to the platform with a universal joint, as shown in Fig. 4. The central strut is used to connect the platform to the base. Each limb consists of a prismatic joint and is attached to the platform with a spherical joint and to the base with a universal joint. Due to the fact that three actuators are used for operating this 2-DOF platform, the mechanism is redundantly actuated.

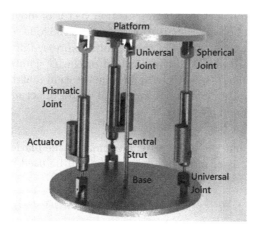

Fig. 4. A CAD model of the redundantly actuated 2-DOF 3-UPS parallel platform.

3.2   Inverse Kinematics of the Platform

The Inverse Kinematical Analysis of a 2-DOF Redundantly actuated 3-UPS Platform has been done by Saglia et al. [7]. For our design, the frame assignments is done as shown in Fig. 5 for developing the Kinematic Model.

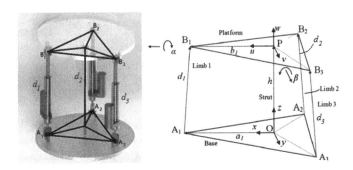

Fig. 5. Geometry of the parallel mechanism and frame assignment for kinematic modelling.

As shown in Fig. 5, two Cartesian coordinate systems $O_{x,y,z}$ as the fixed frame attached to the base and $P_{u,v,w}$ moving reference frame attached to the platform, are chosen, with (x, y, z) and (u, v, w) as the unit vectors of the reference frames O and P, respectively.

Defining two rotation angles α and β as roll and pitch about axes $\boldsymbol{u}$ and $\boldsymbol{v}$, we can describe the orientation of the moving platform with respect to the base frame. Referring to Fig. 5, a loop-closure equation for each limb $\boldsymbol{i}$ in vector form can be written as

$$\overrightarrow{A_i B_i} = \boldsymbol{d_i} = \boldsymbol{p} + \boldsymbol{b_i} - \boldsymbol{a_i} = \boldsymbol{p} + R_P^O \boldsymbol{b_i^P} - \boldsymbol{a_i} \tag{1}$$

where $\boldsymbol{d_i}$ is the ith limb vector, $\boldsymbol{p}$ is the position vector of moving frame origin in base frame, $\boldsymbol{a_i}$, $\boldsymbol{b_i}$ and $\boldsymbol{b_i^P}$ are the position vectors of the joint A_i expressed in the base reference frame, the position of the B_i joint expressed in the platform fixed orientation reference frame, and the position of the B_i joints expressed in the moving reference frame, respectively. R_P^O is the rotation matrix representing the orientation of moving frame in base frame. The vector of actuated joint positions for three limbs is defined as

$$t = [d_1 \ d_2 \ d_3]^T \tag{2}$$

However, finding out the unit vector $\hat{n}$ normal to the platform after it undergoes the rotation R_P^O is of more interest as this will be used in the forthcoming section. The vector $\hat{n}$ is given by

$$\hat{n} = [sin(\beta)cos(\alpha) \ - sin(\alpha) \ cos(\beta)cos(\alpha)] \tag{3}$$

Let $\hat{n} = [n_x n_y n_z]^T$ then,

$$\beta = atan2(n_x, n_z) \tag{4}$$

$$\alpha = atan2(-n_y, (n_x^2 + n_z^2)^{1/2}) \tag{5}$$

4 Algorithm to Calculate the Velocity and Angle of Launch for the Ball

4.1 Terminology and Symbols

Following terminology and symbols are used in the following development:

Ellipse of Points of Maximum Heights ($\hat{E}$). As shown in Fig. 6, the curve joining the points of maximum height in the parabolas of ideal projectile motion can be shown to be an ellipse [2]. This ellipse $\hat{E}$ will be used ahead for formulating the problem its solution method. The equation of this ellipse $\hat{E}$ is given by,

$$\frac{x^2}{a^2} + \frac{(y-b)^2}{b^2} \tag{6}$$

where, $a = \frac{v_0^2}{2g}$, $b = \frac{v_0^2}{2g}$, with v_0 as the magnitude of initial velocity of projectile and g is the acceleration due to gravity.

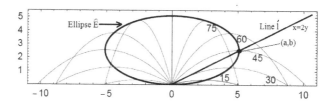

Fig. 6. Ellipse of points of maximum heights [2].

Locus of the Rightmost Points of the Ellipse $\hat{E}$ (Line $\hat{l}$). The rightmost point of the ellipse $\hat{E}$ is (a, b) and as $a = 2b$, the locus of the rightmost points of the family of ellipses $\hat{E}$ is $x = 2y$, which turns out to be a line. This line will be denoted by the symbol $\hat{l}$.

Angle of Launch (θ_k). The angle of launch for any point k lying on the ellipse $\hat{E}$ can be found by the following equations:

$$\theta = \frac{1}{2}\sin^{-1}\left(\frac{2gx}{v_0^2}\right) \text{ when } y < b \tag{7}$$

$$\theta = \frac{\pi}{2} - \frac{1}{2}\sin^{-1}\left(\frac{2gx}{v_0^2}\right) \text{ when } y > b \tag{8}$$

where, x and y are the coordinates of the point k.

4.2   Computation of Ball Velocity and Angle of Launch for High Catches

Every fielder has a maximum area of reach on the field where he can get to and make a catch possible. We define this area as "horizontal circle of maximum reach", a circle with radius R. A catch has been defined as a high catch if the point of maximum height of the balls trajectory is greater than or equal to a user defined value H and falls in the area of maximum reach i.e. a circle of radius R. Figure 7 shows an example of High catch.

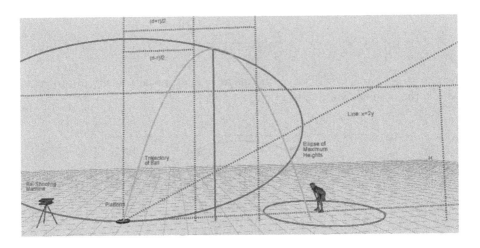

Fig. 7. A high catch geometry.

The aim is to find an appropriate velocity and angle of launch for the ball so that it lands in the horizontal circle of maximum reach.

As shown in Fig. 8, let the line OB formed by the plane of the balls trajectory and the ground make an angle of ϕ with the line OA joining the centre of the platform and the position of the player. The value of ϕ is restricted by the circle of maximum reach in the range $-\sin^{-1}\left(\frac{R}{D}\right)$ and $\sin^{-1}\left(\frac{R}{D}\right)$ where, D is the distance of the fielder from the platform. The distances d and r are given by the following equations:

$$d = \frac{cot(\phi)D}{\sqrt{1 + (cot(\phi))^2}} \tag{9}$$

$$r = \sqrt{R^2 - \frac{D^2}{1 + (cot(\phi))^2}} \tag{10}$$

The solution is developed by restricting the horizontal range of the ball between $d - r$ and $d + r$ (i.e. segment BC) such that the maximum height attained by the ball is greater than or equal to H (Fig. 8). A projectile attains

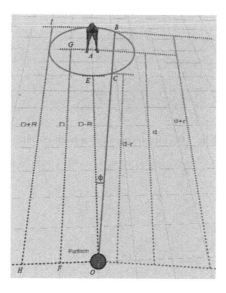

Fig. 8. The projected ball must fall anywhere on the segment BC.

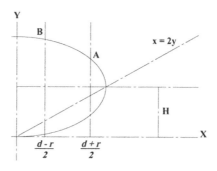

Fig. 9. The segment AB of the ellipse contains the suitable points of maximum heights.

maximum height when it has covered half of its horizontal range. Therefore, the x coordinate of the point of maximum height for the projected ball must lie between the values $p = \frac{d-r}{2}$ and $q = \frac{d+r}{2}$. Figure 9 shows an ellipse $\hat{E}$ drawn for a certain velocity. The segment AB of the ellipse $\hat{E}$ shown in this figure, thus contains the suitable points of maximum height of the trajectory of projected ball.

Three situations are possible for the catch as shown in Fig. 10. Case I has both the points p and q on the left hand side of the line $\hat{l}$, Case II has the line $\hat{l}$ lying between the points p and q and Case III has the points p and q on the right hand side of line $\hat{l}$.

Each case will have an Ellipse $\hat{E}$ corresponding to the minimum velocity v_{min} that satisfies the condition for the range of the ball to lie between $d-r$ and $d+r$

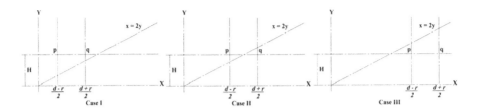

Fig. 10. Three cases for a high catch.

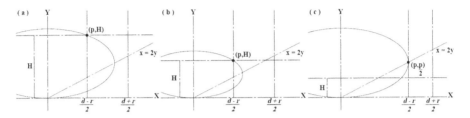

Fig. 11. Ellipse corresponding to the velocity $v_{\min}$. In (a) and (b) passing through (p, H) for Case I and II respectively and in (c) passing through $\left(p, \frac{p}{2}\right)$ for Case III.

and attain maximum height greater than or equal to H. For Case I, this ellipse should pass through the point (p, H) as shown in Fig. 11(a). Substituting this point in the ellipse equation 6 gives the expression for $v_{\min}$ as:

$$v_{min} = \sqrt{\frac{4g(p^2 + 4H^2)}{8H}} \tag{11}$$

The ellipse $\hat{E}$ corresponding to the minimum velocity for Case II also passes through the point (p, H) and the velocity is again given by (11). For Case III, this ellipse passes through the point $\left(p, \frac{p}{2}\right)$ sitting on the line $\hat{l}$ as shown in Fig. 11(c). Substituting this point in (6) gives the following expression for $v_{\min}$

$$v_{min} = \sqrt{2gp} \tag{12}$$

The maximum velocity $v_{\max}$ of the ball is restricted by the Ball Shooting Machine. A random velocity v_0 is chosen between $v_{\min}$ and $v_{\max}$, the ellipse $\hat{E}$ corresponding to this chosen velocity is drawn, suitable segments of this ellipse (as was done in Fig. 9) is found and hence the range of values for the angle of launch which satisfy the conditions required is calculated.

Depending on the distances d, r, H and the chosen velocity v_0, two subcases for Case I, three subcases for Case II and five subcases for Case III arise which are shown in Fig. 12. The segments on each of the ellipse constrained by the region $x \geq \frac{(d-r)}{2}$, $x \leq \frac{(d-r)}{2}$ and $y \geq H$, contain the suitable points of maximum height. A range of values for the angle of launch is calculated for each case and a random angle θ is selected from this range.

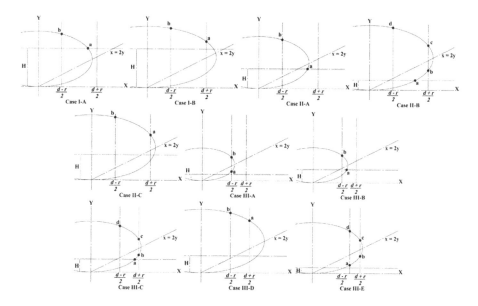

Fig. 12. Subcases for Case I, Case II and Case III of high catches

For example, for Case III-C in Fig. 12,

$$\theta_1 = random(\theta_a, \theta_b) \tag{13}$$

$$\theta_2 = random(\theta_c, \theta_d) \tag{14}$$

$$\theta = random(\theta_1, \theta_2) \tag{15}$$

where, the function $random(s,t)$ returns a random value between the values s and t.

4.3   Computation of Ball Velocity and Angle of Launch for Flat Catches

As their name suggests, flat catches are the ones which are hit hard and follow flat trajectories. The definition used for a flat catch is similar to that of the high catch except that the point of maximum height of the ball's trajectory is less than or equal to a user defined value H. Figure 13 shows an example of a flat catch. The solution methodology to find the velocity and angle of launch for the ball to provide a flat catch is similar to that used for providing a high catch. As in the case of high catch, cases similar to the ones shown in the Fig. 10 arise.

Each case will have an Ellipse $\hat{E}$ corresponding to the minimum velocity v_{min} that satisfies the condition for the range of the ball to lie between $d-r$ and $d+r$ and attain a minimum height less than or equal to H. For Case I, this ellipse should pass through the point $\left(p, \frac{p}{2}\right)$ as shown in Fig. 14(a). Substituting this point in the ellipse equation (6) gives the expression for v_{min} as:

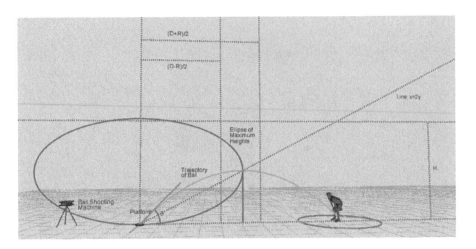

Fig. 13. A flat catch geometry.

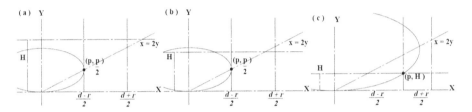

Fig. 14. Ellipse corresponding to the velocity v_{min}. In (a) and (b) passing through $\left(p, \frac{p}{2}\right)$ for Case I and II respectively and in (c) passing through (p, H) for Case III.

$$v_{min} = \sqrt{2gp} \tag{16}$$

The ellipse $\hat{E}$ corresponding to the minimum velocity for Case II also passes through the point $\left(p, \frac{p}{2}\right)$ and the velocity is again given by (11). For Case III, this ellipse passes through the point (p, H) sitting on the line H as shown in Fig. 14(c). Substituting this point in (6) gives the following expression for v_{min}

$$v_{min} = \sqrt{\frac{4g(p^2 + 4H^2)}{8H}} \tag{17}$$

The maximum velocity v_{max} of the ball is restricted by the Ball Shooting Machine. A random velocity v_0 is chosen between v_{min} and v_{max}, the ellipse $\hat{E}$ corresponding to this chosen velocity is drawn, suitable segments of this ellipse (as was done in Fig. 9) is found and hence the range of values for the angle of launch which satisfy the conditions required is calculated.

Depending on the distances d, r, H and the chosen velocity v_0, five subcases for Case I, three subcases for Case II and two subcases for Case III arise which

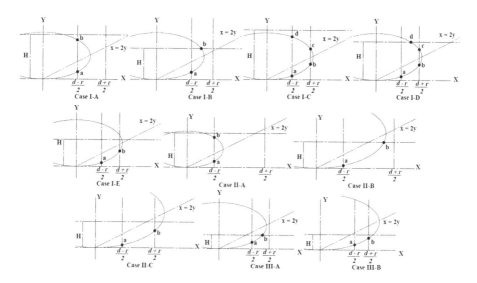

Fig. 15. Subcases for Case I, Case II and Case III of flat catches.

are shown in Fig. 15. The segments on each of the ellipse constrained by the region $x \geq \frac{(d-r)}{2}$, $x \leq \frac{(d-r)}{2}$ and $y \leq H$, contain the suitable points of maximum height. A range of values for the angle of launch is calculated for each case and a random angle θ is selected from this range.

4.4   Computation of Ball Velocity and Angle of Launch for Reaction Catches

Most commonly, catches in Cricket are taken close to the wicket. The catches taken in slips, at short leg or silly point are often reaction catches. These catches have a very less reaction time, usually ranging from 0.5 s to 1.5 s. This time is not enough for the player to move horizontally on the ground and thus, here, the fielder won't have a horizontal circle of maximum reach. We formulate the problem of providing reaction catches by having a "diving semicircle of maximum reach" as shown the Fig. 16. The ball after being swerved by the platform must pass through this semicircle, and an appropriate velocity and angle of launch is calculated to accomplish this task.

As shown in Fig. 17, let the line OB formed by the plane of the balls trajectory and the ground make an angle of ϕ with the line OA joining the centre of the platform and the position of the player. The value of ϕ is restricted by the diving semicircle of maximum reach in the range $-\tan^{-1}\left(\frac{H}{D}\right)$ and $\tan^{-1}\left(\frac{H}{D}\right)$ where, D is the distance of the fielder from the platform and H is the radius of the diving semicircle. The distances d and h are given by the following equations:

$$d = \frac{D}{cos(\phi)} \tag{18}$$

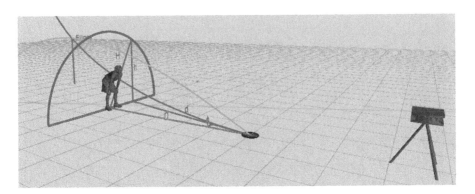

Fig. 16. A reaction catch geometry.

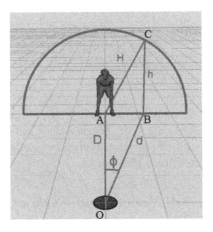

Fig. 17. The projected ball must pass through the segment BC.

$$h = \sqrt{H^2 - (Dtan(\phi))^2} \qquad (19)$$

As discussed earlier, the reaction time in case of a reaction catch ranges from 0.5 s to 1.5 s. To calculate the velocity v and angle of launch θ, we set the trajectory of the ball such that the ball reaches the segment BC in a random time t in the range of 0.5 s to 1.5 s and at a random point on the segment BC at a height of p from the ground. Thus, $t \in [0.5, 1.5]$ and $p \in [0, h]$. This provides the following equations for the velocity and angle of launch for the ball:

$$\theta = \tan^{-1}\left(\frac{p + \frac{1}{2}gt^2}{d}\right) \qquad (20)$$

$$v = \frac{p + \frac{1}{2}gt^2}{tsin(\theta)} \qquad (21)$$

5   Velocity and Angle of Launch of the Ball Shot from Ball Shooting Machine

In case a Ball Shooting Machine is used, the velocity and angle of launch of the ball needs to be calculated so that the ball hits the center of the platform and finally drops in the desired radius of maximum reach of the fielder. As shown in Fig. 18, let the Ball Shooting Machine be placed at a distance A from the platform and the ball be shot from a height of B from the ground. If v_0 is the required velocity of launch as the ball leaves the platform after hitting it, then the velocity of launch v_b from the Ball Shooting Machine is given by the expression

$$v_b = \sqrt{v_0^2 - 2gB} \tag{22}$$

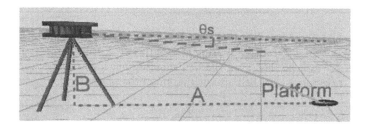

Fig. 18. Trajectory of the ball shot from the ball shooting machine onto the platform.

The angle of launch θ_s can be found from the expression

$$\theta_s = \tan^{-1}\left(\frac{-A + \sqrt{A^2 - 2\left(\frac{gA^2}{v_b^2}\right)\left(\frac{gA^2}{2v_b^2} - B\right)}}{\left(\frac{gA^2}{v_b^2}\right)}\right) \tag{23}$$

6   Orientation of the Platform

The orientation of the platform to swerve the ball shot from the ball shooting machine is computed as follows. If v_{in} is the velocity vector of the ball just before striking the platform and v_{out} the velocity vector just after striking the platform, then the unit vector normal to the platform $\hat{n}$ can given as:

$$\hat{n} = norm(\overrightarrow{v_{out}} - \overrightarrow{v_{in}}) \tag{24}$$

where, *norm* provides a normalized vector. Equations (2–5) along with (24) can be used to calculate vector of actuated joint positions of three limbs supporting the platform $t = [d_1 \ d_2 \ d_3]^T$.

7 Simulation Results

The simulation of the proposed system was done in an Open-Source Software, *Processing* [6]. The simulation results for High Catches launched at various speeds and launch angles are shown in the Figs. (19, 20 and 21). For all the simulations, the maximum velocity of launch for the ball that can be provided is constrained by the Ball Shooting machine and is taken as $30\,\mathrm{ms}^{-1}$. Figure 19

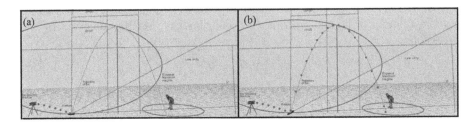

Fig. 19. Screenshots of simulation of a high catch with launch velocity of $13\,\mathrm{ms}^{-1}$, angle of launch $\theta = 1.30\,\mathrm{rad}$, $H = 6\,\mathrm{m}$, $D = 10\,\mathrm{m}$, $R = 3\,\mathrm{m}$ and $\phi = 0.2\,\mathrm{rad}$. (a) Trajectory of the ball as shot from the ball shooting machine towards the platform. (b) Swerved trajectory of the ball after actuation of the platform.

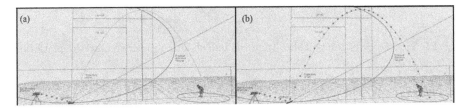

Fig. 20. Screenshots of simulation of a high catch with launch velocity of $15\,\mathrm{ms}^{-1}$, angle of launch $\theta = 1.19\,\mathrm{rad}$, $H = 3.5\,\mathrm{m}$, $D = 15\,\mathrm{m}$, $R = 3\,\mathrm{m}$ and $\phi = 0.079\,\mathrm{rad}$. (a) Trajectory of the ball as shot from the Ball Shooting Machine towards the platform. (b) Swerved trajectory of the ball after actuation of the platform.

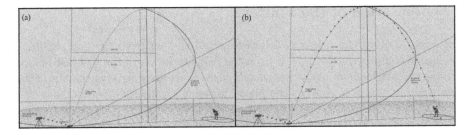

Fig. 21. Screenshots of simulation of a high catch with launch velocity of $18\,\mathrm{ms}^{-1}$, angle of launch $\theta = 1.25\,\mathrm{rad}$, $H = 3\,\mathrm{m}$, $D = 20\,\mathrm{m}$, $R = 2\,\mathrm{m}$ and $\phi = 0.059\,\mathrm{rad}$. (a) Trajectory of the ball as shot from the ball shooting machine towards the platform. (b) Swerved trajectory of the ball after actuation of the platform.

shows an example of the Case I-B for a High Catch. In this example, the parameters D, R, ϕ and H have the values 10 m, 3 m, 0.2 rad and 6 m respectively. The minimum velocity of launch for this case can be found using (11). This provides a range from $11.36\,\text{ms}^{-1}$ to $30\,\text{ms}^{-1}$ for choosing the velocity of launch for the ball. In this example, the velocity of launch was chosen as $13.00\,\text{ms}^{-1}$. This chosen velocity in turn provides a range from 1.184 rad to 1.344 rad for the angle of launch. In this example, the angle of launch was chosen as 1.30 rad. Figures 20

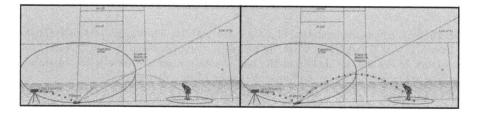

Fig. 22. Screenshots of simulation of a flat catch with launch velocity of $10\,\text{ms}^{-1}$, angle of launch $\theta = 0.756\,\text{rad}$, $H = 5\,\text{m}$, $D = 10\,\text{m}$, $R = 2\,\text{m}$ and $\phi = 0.09\,\text{rad}$. (a) Trajectory of the ball as shot from the ball shooting machine towards the platform. (b) Swerved trajectory of the ball after actuation of the platform.

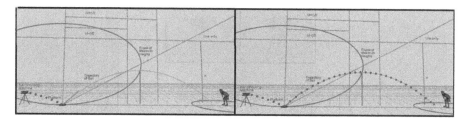

Fig. 23. Screenshots of simulation of a flat catch with launch velocity of $12\,\text{ms}^{-1}$, angle of launch $\theta = 0.6995\,\text{rad}$, $H = 6\,\text{m}$, $D = 15\,\text{m}$, $R = 3\,\text{m}$ and $\phi = -0.10067\,\text{rad}$. (a) Trajectory of the ball as shot from the ball shooting machine towards the platform. (b) Swerved trajectory of the ball after actuation of the platform.

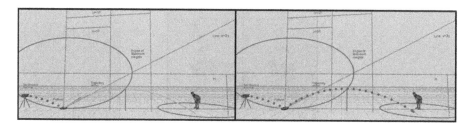

Fig. 24. Screenshots of simulation of a flat catch with launch velocity of $11\,\text{ms}^{-1}$, angle of launch $\theta = 0.5665\,\text{rad}$, $H = 3\,\text{m}$, $D = 12\,\text{m}$, $R = 3.5\,\text{m}$ and $\phi = -0.1215\,\text{rad}$. (a) Trajectory of the ball as shot from the ball shooting machine towards the platform. (b) Swerved trajectory of the ball after actuation of the platform.

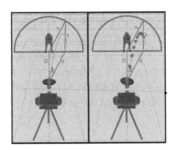

Fig. 25. Screenshots of simulation of a flat catch with launch velocity of $8\,\mathrm{ms}^{-1}$, angle of launch $\theta = 0.77\,\mathrm{rad}$, $H = 2.5\,\mathrm{m}$, $D = 5\,\mathrm{m}$, $t = 0.8705\,\mathrm{s}$ and $\phi = 0.2318\,\mathrm{rad}$. (a) Trajectory of the ball as shot from the ball shooting machine towards the platform. (b) Swerved trajectory of the ball after actuation of the platform.

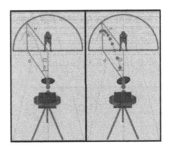

Fig. 26. Screenshots of simulation of a flat catch with launch velocity of $9.056\,\mathrm{ms}^{-1}$, angle of launch $\theta = 0.6502\,\mathrm{rad}$, $H = 2.5\,\mathrm{m}$, $D = 5\,\mathrm{m}$, $t = 0.7238\,\mathrm{s}$ and $\phi = -0.29\,\mathrm{rad}$. (a) Trajectory of the ball as shot from the ball shooting machine towards the platform. (b) Swerved trajectory of the ball after actuation of the platform.

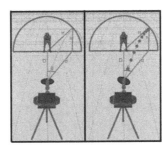

Fig. 27. Screenshots of simulation of a flat catch with launch velocity of $1.0056\,\mathrm{ms}^{-1}$, angle of launch $\theta = 0.578\,\mathrm{rad}$, $H = 2.5\,\mathrm{m}$, $D = 5\,\mathrm{m}$, $t = 0.6319\,\mathrm{s}$ and $\phi = 0.35\,\mathrm{rad}$. (a) Trajectory of the ball as shot from the ball shooting machine towards the platform. (b) Swerved trajectory of the ball after actuation of the platform.

and 21 are the examples of Case II-C and Case III-D respectively. Similarly, Figs. (22, 23 and 24) show simulation results for Flat Catches and Figs. (25, 26 and 27) show the simulation of reaction catches, launched at various velocities and launch angles.

These simulation results prove the idea that the proposed 2-DOF 3-UPS Parallel Platform can be very effectively used for catching practice drills in Cricket and can be used to train the players for their weak points. The platform is being fabricated to perform field trials.

8   Conclusion and Further Work

High, Flat and Reaction catches are the three common types of catches a fielder encounters in Cricket. Our previous work [1] focussed on the formulation of a methodology to provide catching practice for High catches. This work extends our previous work by formulating methodologies to provide catching practice for Flat and Reaction catches. The formulation methodology for providing Flat catches is quite similar to that for the High catches, due to similarities in their problem definitions. Formulation methodology for providing Reaction catches is different from that for the High and Flat catches, as in this case, we have a diving semicircle of maximum reach instead of a horizontal circle of maximum reach, due to less reaction time.

Our proposed platform and methodology is capable of providing catching drills while maintaining a degree of realism. The proposed technique can be easily adapted for training players for many other sports including baseball. It can also be used for training sports-persons and players for developing their visual tracking skills, reaction skills, and catching skills.

Air drag, wind velocity and other effects can deviate a projectile from its actual parabolic trajectory. In realistic situation, the ball shot from the Ball Shooting Machine may not hit the center of the platform due to these unconsidered effects. Our future work will address this problem by making use of a 5-DOF (3 translational and 2 rotational) architecture for the platform. The trajectory of the ball will be tracked and predicted by adopting Visual Servoing techniques to control the 5-DOF platform in real-time.

Regrettably, this platform is incapable of simulating aspects, related to body position/movement of the batsman and tackling this problem will also form a part in the future work of this project.

References

1. Bhole, A.A., Mittal, R.K.: Cricket catching drills - application of a redundantly actuated 2-DOF 3-UPS parallel platform to increase the efficacy of providing catching practice drills in cricket. In: Proceedings of the 3rd International Congress on Sport Sciences Research and Technology Support, pp. 190–197 (2015)
2. Fernández-Chapou, J., Salas-Brito, A., Vargas, C.: An elliptic property of parabolic trajectories. arXiv preprint physics/0402020 (2004)

3. Mecademic: What is a parallel robot? (2013). http://www.mecademic.com/What-is-a-parallel-robot.html
4. Morgan, E.: Eoin morgan unbelievable shot in the big bash! (2014). https://www.youtube.com/watch?v=IC_lbWUZlsA
5. Muller, A.: Parallel Manipulators - Towards New Applications. I-Tech Education and Publishing, Wien (2008)
6. Processing: Processing.org (2001). https://processing.org/
7. Saglia, J.A., Dai, J.S., Caldwell, D.G.: Geometry and kinematic analysis of a redundantly actuated parallel mechanism that eliminates singularities and improves dexterity. J. Mech. Des. **130**(12), 124–501 (2008)

Design Optimization of the Landing Slope of a Ski Jumping Hill

Kazuya Seo[1(✉)], Yuji Nihei[2], Toshiyuki Shimano[3], and Yuji Ohgi[4]

[1] Yamagata University, 1-4-12 Kojirakawa, Yamagata, Japan
seo@e.yamagata-u.ac.jp
[2] Yamagata City Office, 2-3-25 Hatagomachi, Yamagata, Japan
[3] Access Corporation, 2-3-4, Minami-1-jo Higashi, Chuo-ku, Sapporo, Japan
[4] Keio University, 5322 Endo, Fujisawa, Japan

Abstract. This paper describes a procedure for optimizing the design of the landing slope of the Zao jumping hill. The concept behind the design of the landing slope is that the landing slope should enable the spectators to witness an exciting spectacle, that the jumpers can land safely, and that it can be constructed with minimum cost. We regard these features as objective functions. The findings can be summarized as follows: it is possible to control the objective functions by changing the profile of the landing slope; there is not a unique optimal design solution, but the Pareto optimal solutions; a landing slope that gives safety on landing is almost equivalent to a landing slope that produces differences in the flight distance due to differences the jumpers' skill levels; there is a trade-off between the length of the flight distance and safety on landing; the construction cost is influenced by the horizontal distance between the edge of the take-off table and the K-point. The developed procedure would be applicable not only to Zao in Yamagata city, but also to all ski jumping hills in the world.

Keywords: Optimal design · Flight simulation · Ski jumping · Landing slope · Exciting spectacle · Safety landing Construction cost

Nomenclature

b	Width of the landing slope
D	Drag
FD_i	Flight distance around the local longest flight distance, FD_L
FD_L	The local longest flight distance
$F1$	The first objective function, construction cost
$F2$	The second objective function, landing velocity
$F3$	The third objective function, flight distance multiplied by -1
$F4$	The forth objective function, standard deviation in flight distance due to differences in the jumpers' skill levels
g	Gravitational acceleration
H	Height difference between the old Zao and the new Zao
h	Height difference between the edge of the take-off table and the K-point of the landing slope
I_{yy}	Moment of inertia of the body–ski combination on its y_b–axis
L	Lift

© Springer International Publishing AG 2016
J. Cabri and P. Pezarat Correia (Eds.): icSPORTS 2015, CCIS 632, pp. 57–70, 2016.
DOI: 10.1007/978-3-319-52770-3_5

M	Pitching moment
m	Mass of the body–ski combination
N	Number of Monte-Carlo simulations
n	Horizontal distance between the edge of the take-off table and the K-point of the landing slope
Q	Y_b component of the angular velocity vector
r_L	Radius of the landing area curve
r_{2L}	Radius of the transition curve from L to U at L
r_2	Radius of the transition curve from L to U at U
t_f	Flight time
(U,W)	(x_b, z_b) components of the velocity vector
V	Amplitude of the velocity vector of the ski jumper
$v_\perp$	Landing velocity, velocity component of the ski jumper perpendicular to the landing slope at the point of landing
(X_a, Z_a)	(x_b, z_b) components of the aerodynamic force
(x_b, z_b)	Body-fixed coordinate system
(X_E, Z_E)	Inertial coordinate system
Z_N	Vertical position of the new Zao at X_E
Z_O	Vertical position of the old Zao at X_E
Z_U	Bottom of the landing slope of the old Zao
α	Angle of attack
β	Forward leaning angle
β_k	Slope of the landing hill at the K-point
β_H	Slope of the landing hill at the landing position
γ	Flight path angle
λ	Ski-opening angle
Θ	Pitch angle

1 Introduction

Since 2012 the Zao jumping hill in Yamagata city has been host to the annual ladies world cup. A ski jumping hill is composed of the in-run, the take-off table, the landing slope and the out-run. The Zao track was renovated to resemble the ski jump at the Sochi Games in 2013, with a take-off table with an angle of 11° downhill. A further renovation related to the landing slope is being planned for 2015, and this is the subject of this study. It is likely to cost 700,000,000 Japanese yen (5,800,000 USD, or 5,000,000 EUR), so there is a huge responsibility on the shoulders of the authors.

The concept behind the design of the landing slope is that the landing slope should enable the spectators to witness an exciting spectacle, that the jumpers should land safely, and that it can be constructed with the minimum cost. These concepts were converted to the values of four objective functions.

2 Flight Simulation

In order to estimate objective functions in Sect. 3, the flight trajectory needs to be simulated. The flight trajectory is obtained by integrating the equations of motion.

It is assumed that the motion of the body–ski combination occurs in a fixed vertical plane. The coordinate systems and the definitions of the characteristic parameters are shown in Fig. 1. The origin of the inertial coordinate system (X_E, Z_E) is defined as being at the edge of the take-off table, while the X_E-axis is in the horizontal forward direction and the Z_E-axis is vertically downward. On the other hand, the origin of the body-fixed coordinate system (x_b, z_b) is defined as the center of gravity of the body–ski combination.

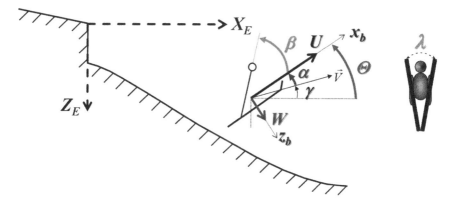

Fig. 1. Coordinate systems and definition of characteristic parameters.

In terms of coordinate transformations in a fixed vertical plane we then have

$$\dot{X}_E = U \cos \Theta + W \sin \Theta \tag{1}$$

$$\dot{Z}_E = -U \sin \Theta + W \cos \Theta \tag{2}$$

Here, (U, W) are the (x_b, z_b) components of the velocity vector. The equations of motion and the moment equation are

$$\dot{U} = \frac{1}{m}[X_a - mg \sin \Theta] - QW \tag{3}$$

$$\dot{W} = \frac{1}{m}[Z_a + mg \cos \Theta] + QU \tag{4}$$

$$\dot{Q} = \frac{M_a}{I_{yy}} \tag{5}$$

$$\dot{\Theta} = Q \tag{6}$$

Here, (X_a, Z_a) are the (x_b, z_b) components of the aerodynamic force, Q is the y_b component of the angular velocity vector, m is the mass of the body–ski combination, g is the gravitational acceleration, M_a is the y_b component of the aerodynamic moment, and I_{yy} is the moment of inertia of the body–ski combination on the y_b-axis. The flight trajectory $(X_E(t), Y_E(t))$ can be obtained by integrating Eq. (1) through (6) numerically.

The aerodynamic forces X_a and Z_a in Eqs. (3) and (4) are derived from D and L as given in Eqs. (7) and (8).

$$X_a = L \sin \alpha - D \cos \alpha \tag{7}$$

$$Z_a = -L \cos \alpha - D \sin \alpha \tag{8}$$

The aerodynamic drag, lift and moment in Eq. (3) through (5) were all obtained during wind tunnel tests as functions of α, β and λ [1]. The wind tunnel data were acquired for α at 5° intervals between 0° and 40°, and for β at intervals of 10° between 0° and 40°, respectively. The ski-opening angle λ was set at one of 0°, 10° and 25°. The torso and legs of the model were always set in a straight line. The tails of the skis were always in contact on the inner edges.

3 Objective Functions

The construction cost was estimated on the basis of the amount of material that is needed to construct the new slope. Some of this material will be moved from the existing Zao jumping hill, while new material will also have to be brought in. Lower cost is, of course, better.

The safety on landing was estimated on the basis of the landing velocity [2]. The landing velocity is the velocity component perpendicular to the landing slope at the instance of landing, and this needs to be small to reduce the impact and make the landing safer.

A long flight distance provides an exciting spectacle for the spectators. The first objective function for the Zao jumping hill is the flight distance; the longer the flight distance, the more exciting the spectacle.

On the other hand, the landing slope in Zao is designed to make the differences in the flight distance greater with respect to differences in the skill-levels of the jumpers. The flight distances could be maximized if jumpers were able to satisfy the optimal conditions from take-off through to landing. However, less-skilled jumpers are unable to satisfy the optimal conditions during every flight. This shortens the flight distance. One of the design objectives in Zao is to enhance this variance in the flight distance. In other words, the jumpers should control their attitude correctly every flight in order to win at the Zao jumping hill. A skilled jumper who can control their attitude correctly every flight can win at Zao. The greater the variance of the flight distance due to the skill difference, the more exciting the spectacle. The second objective function is the standard deviation in the flight distance due to the jumper's skill difference.

In order to estimate the values of the objective functions, the flight trajectory needs to be simulated. This has already been discussed in Sect. 2.

3.1   Construction Cost

The construction cost was estimated on the basis of the amount of material needed to construct the new slope. This is the first objective function, $F1$.

The height difference between the old Zao and the new Zao at X_E is denoted by H (X_E) in Eq. (9).

$$H(X_E) = Z_N(X_E) - Z_O(X_E) \tag{9}$$

Here, the height of the new landing slope is denoted by Z_N, while that of the old landing slope is denoted by Z_O.

The width of the new landing slope at X_E is denoted by $b(X_E)$. The amount of material needed to construct the new jumping hill is derived using Eq. (10).

$$\text{Amount of material} = \int_0^{132} |H(X_E)| \cdot b(X_E) \, dX_E \tag{10}$$

Here, the value of 132 is the X_E value at the bottom of the slope, Z_U.

The construction cost depends on the height to which material needs to be taken to construct the new hill. The greater the height, the more expensive the construction cost. Here, the lowest cost is at Z_U and this is assumed to be 200 Japanese yen per 1 m³, while the highest cost is at $Z_E = 0$ (at the top of the slope), which is assumed to be 10,000 yen per 1 m³ on the basis of experience. The cost between Z_U and $Z_E = 0$ is derived using a linear relationship between cost and height. Therefore, the construction cost, $F1$, can be estimated using Eq. (11).

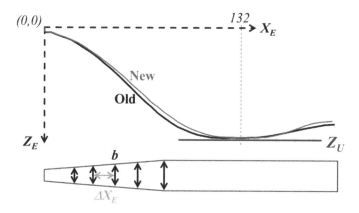

Fig. 2. The schematic of the landing profiles of the new and old Zao. The new Zao is denoted by the red line, while that of the old Zao is denoted by the black line. (Color figure online)

$$F1 = \int_0^{132} |H(X_E)| \cdot b(X_E) \cdot \left\{ -\frac{9800}{Z_U}(Z_O(X_E) - Z_U) + 200 \right\} dX_E \qquad (11)$$

3.2 Safety Landing

The safety on landing was estimated on the basis of the landing velocity. The landing velocity is the velocity component perpendicular to the landing slope at the instance of

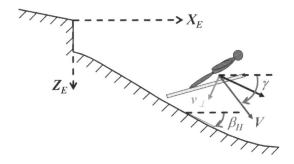

Fig. 3. Landing velocity, $v\perp$, which is the velocity component perpendicular to the landing slope at the point of landing.

landing (Fig. 3), and this needs to be small to reduce the impact and make the landing safer. The landing velocity, $F2$, is shown in Eq. (12), where the flight path angle and the slope of the landing hill at the landing point are denoted by γ and β_H.

$$F2 = v_\perp = V \sin(\gamma - \beta_H) \qquad (12)$$

3.3 Flight Distance

A ski jumping hill should be designed so that it contributes to the creation of an exciting spectacle, which means that the jumpers have longer flight distances. The flight distance is defined by the distance along the profile of the landing slope. $F3$, which is the flight distance multiplied by –1, is obtained from Eq. (13). Here, the flight time is denoted by t_f.

$$F3 = -\int_0^{X_E(t_f)} \sqrt{1 + \left(\frac{dZ_N}{dX_E}\right)^2} \, dX_E \qquad (13)$$

3.4   Standard Deviation in the Flight Distance Due to the Jumper's Skill Difference

The standard deviation in the flight distance multiplied by −1, *F4*, is defined by Eq. (14), where FD_L is the local longest flight distance, shown by × in Fig. 4, FD_i are the simulated flight distances around FD_L, shown by •, and *N* is the number of flight simulations. The abscissa and the ordinate in Fig. 4 are design variables, which are the angles given in #7 through #22 in Table 1 in Sect. 4. The ellipse in Fig. 4 corresponds to the human error. Since the jumper is not a robot, there will be some human error, which shortens the flight distance. The human error is assumed to be 2° for all angles

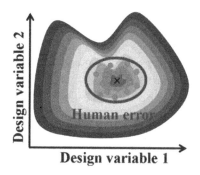

Fig. 4.   Contour map of flight distance. FD_L: Longest flight distance shown by ×, FD_i: Flight distances around FD_L shown by •.

from #7 through #22. Fifty Monte-Carlo simulations of the flight distance around FD_L in the range for human errors of 2° were carried out 50 times (*N* = 50). These fifty simulations produce fifty FD_is, therefore the standard deviation of the flight distance, *F4*, can be estimated by Eq. (14).

$$F4 = -\sqrt{\frac{\sum_{i=1}^{N}(FD_i - FD_L)^2}{N-1}} \tag{14}$$

4   Design Variables

The 22 design variables are shown in Table 1. The first six are concerned with the landing slope (Fig. 5), while the other 16 are concerned with various angles of the jumper during the jump. The horizontal and vertical distances between the edge of the take-off table and the K-point are denoted by *n* and *h*. The radii of the landing area curve, the transition curve from L to U at L, and the transition curve from L to U at U are denoted by r_L, r_{2L} and r_2, respectively.

Table 1. Design variables.

#	Design variables	Ranges for GA
1	n	$70 \sim 90$ m
2	β_k	$30 \sim 35°$
3	r_L	$200 \sim 240$ m
4	r_2	$80 \sim 100$ m
5	r_{2L}	$80 \sim 100$ m
6	h/n	$0.541 \sim 0.543$
7	Θ_0	$-11 \sim 10°$
8	Q_0	$-40 \sim 10°/s$
9	β at 0.3 s	$-20 \sim 38°$
10	β at 1.3 s	$2 \sim 38°$
11	β at 2.3 s	$2 \sim 38°$
12	β at 3.3 s	$2 \sim 38°$
13	β at 4.3 s	$2 \sim 38°$
14	β at 5.3 s	$2 \sim 38°$
15	β at 6.3 s	$2 \sim 38°$
16	λ at 0.3 s	$2 \sim 28°$
17	λ at 1.3 s	$2 \sim 28°$
18	λ at 2.3 s	$2 \sim 28°$
19	λ at 3.3 s	$2 \sim 28°$
20	λ at 4.3 s	$2 \sim 28°$
21	λ at 5.3 s	$2 \sim 28°$
22	λ at 6.3 s	$2 \sim 28°$

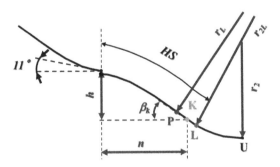

Fig. 5. Landing slope and design variables.

On the other hand, the other 16 are control variables for the jumper. The initial pitch angle is denoted by Θ_0, and the initial angular velocity is denoted by Q_0. The time variations of the forward leaning angle, β, and the ski-opening angle, λ, in Fig. 1 are estimated on the basis of the spline curves, which are constructed from the control points, #9 through 22, in Table 1.

5   Constraints

The take-off table is at an angle of 11° downhill, and the hill size (HS) is set at 106 m (Fig. 5), following a request from Yamagata City Hall. The mass of the body-ski combination is assumed to be 50 kg (female jumpers were assumed), the take-off speed along and perpendicular to the take-off table are assumed to be 24.55 m/s and 2 m/s, respectively. Since there are no experimental aerodynamic data for the high values of β that correspond to the posture in the initial flight phase immediately after take-off, the calculation must begin at 0.3 s after take-off in the present computation. It has been reported that it takes between 0.3 and 0.4 s after take-off to transfer to a stable flight regime [3].

Due to financial reasons, the amount of material needed to reconstruct the Zao jumping hill was limited to

- less than 1.0 m at $X_E = 45$
- less than 2.0 m at $X_E = 80$
- less than 2.0 m at $X_E = 132$ (old U point, in Fig. 5)

Moreover, α, β and λ (Fig. 1) were limited by the experimental ranges, as follows.

- $0° < \alpha < 40°$
- $0° < \beta < 40°$
- $0° < \lambda < 30°$

Although the value of h/n for the old Zao was 0.555, it was limited to between 0.541 and 0.543 in order to adjust the standards for the construction of Jumping Hills [4].

Finally, only flight distances of more than 84 m were considered.

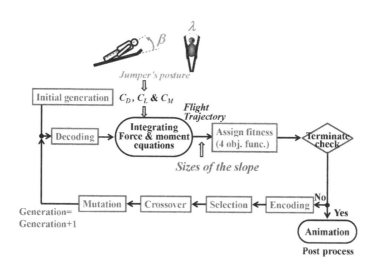

Fig. 6. Genetic algorithm.

6 Optimization

Optimization was carried out with the aid of a genetic algorithm (GA) [5]. A block diagram of the GA is shown in Fig. 6. The GA is a search heuristic that mimics the process of natural selection, so that there are selection, crossover and mutation. Now, there are four objective functions. In order to assign the fitness of the four objective functions, it is necessary to simulate the flight trajectory, which has been discussed in Sect. 2.

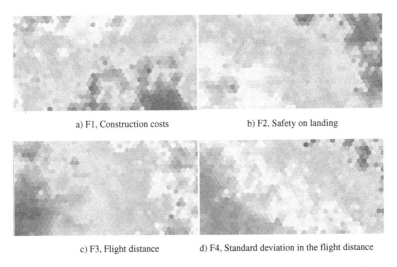

a) F1, Construction costs   b) F2, Safety on landing

c) F3, Flight distance   d) F4, Standard deviation in the flight distance

Fig. 7. Self-organizing maps of the objective functions. (Color figure online)

The 'ranges for GA', which are also shown in Table 1, are defined such that they cover practical values and design regulations. In the optimization process, all the objective functions, from $F1$ through $F4$, in Eq. (11) through (14) should be minimized. The optimization is to determine which set of design variables minimizes all of the objective functions.

7 Results and Discussions

Self-organizing maps (SOM) of the objective functions are shown in Fig. 7. These are contour maps colored by each objective function value. Blue denotes the lowest value, while red denotes the highest. A SOM is useful for enabling low-dimensional views of high-dimensional data [6].

It can be seen from Figs. 7(b) and (d) that the color patterns of the contour maps are almost the same. Therefore, it can be concluded that the safety on landing ($F2$) is almost equivalent to the standard deviation in the flight distance due to the jumper's skill difference ($F4$). The flight trajectory in the extreme optimal solution of $F4$ is

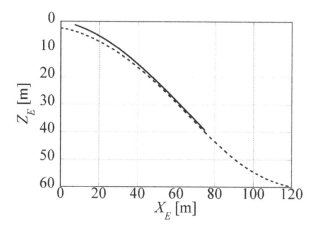

Fig. 8. The flight trajectory and the landing slope in the case of the extreme optimal solution of the greatest standard deviation in the flight distance due to the jumpers' skill differences, *F4*.

shown in Fig. 8. The flight trajectory is denoted by the solid line, while the landing slope is denoted by the broken line. Since the gradient of the landing slope at the landing point is almost parallel to that of the flight trajectory of the jumper, the landing position (therefore, the flight distance) is very sensitive with respect to the jumper's flight control (jumper's skill). Therefore, the same gradient for the flight trajectory and the landing slope at the point of landing gives a larger standard deviation in flight distance. On the other hand, the safest landing is where the gradient of the landing slope at the landing point is almost parallel to that of the flight trajectory of the jumper because the landing velocity, $v_\perp$, becomes the smallest. This is the reason why the safety on landing (*F2*) is almost equivalent to the standard deviation in the flight distance due to differences in the jumpers' skill (*F4*).

The broken line in Fig. 8 is employed by Yamagata city to design a new Zao jumping hill.

The contour maps in Figs. 7(b) and 7(d) are almost the converse of that in Fig. 7(c). This means that there is a trade-off between the flight distance (Fig. 7c) and the other two objective functions (Figs. 7(b) and (d)). Although the lowest values for all the objective functions give the ideal situation, it is impossible to meet this criterion. This is because the four objective functions conflict with one another. The extreme case of the longest flight distance is located at the bottom left hand side of the SOM, where Fig. 7(c) shows the lowest value, and Figs. 7(b) and (d) show almost their highest values. The landing slope that produces the longest flight distance gives the worst safety on landing (dangerous landing) and is the most difficult for unskilled jumpers (the greatest standard deviation in the flight distance due to the jumpers' skill differences).

The contour map of Fig. 7(a) is completely different from the other three maps (Figs. 7(b), (c) and (d)). The color gradient of Fig. 7(a) is in the transverse direction, while the color gradients of the other three maps are in the lateral direction.

Two extreme optimal solutions for the landing slopes are shown in Fig. 9. The broken line shows the profile of the old Zao landing slope, the dash-dot line shows the profile of the lowest cost (opt of *F1*) and the solid line shows the profile of the longest

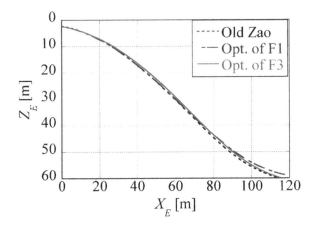

Fig. 9. Comparison between the old Zao landing slope and two extreme optimal solutions of *F1* and *F3*.

flight distance (opt. of *F3*). It is possible to control the construction costs, the flight distance and so on, by changing the profile of the landing slope. The profile of the low cost slope coincides with the old profile, especially at greater height from $Z_E = 0$ through $Z_E = 30$.

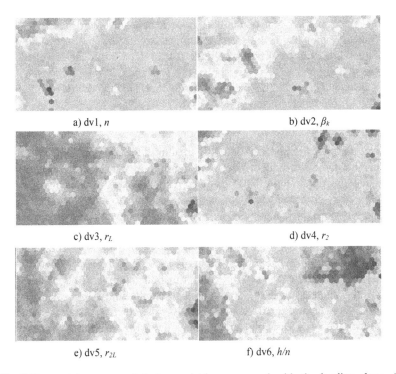

a) dv1, n

b) dv2, β_k

c) dv3, r_L

d) dv4, r_2

e) dv5, r_{2L}

f) dv6, h/n

Fig. 10. Self-organizing maps of design variables concerned with the landing slope. (Color figure online)

The profile which produces the longest flight distances (opt. of $F3$) is higher than that of the lowest cost at $X_E = 40$, while it is lower at $X_E = 90$. Since the flight distance is defined by the distance along the profile, as given by Eq. (13), the profile of the solid line produces longer flight distances for the same trajectory (the same landing position).

Self-organizing maps for the 6 design variables concerned with the landing slope are shown in Fig. 10. It can be seen that the color pattern of Fig. 10(f) is almost the same as those of Figs. 7(b) and (d), while it is almost the converse of that in Fig. 7(c). This means that the three objective functions, $F2$, $F3$ and $F4$ are influenced by h/n. It is self-evident that the smaller h/n makes the flight distance shorter, and vice versa.

The color gradient of Fig. 10(a), n, is in the transverse direction, as in Fig. 7(a). This means that $F1$ is influenced by n.

The color patterns of the other four design variables in Fig. 10 do not match those in Fig. 7. Therefore, these four design variables, β_k, r_L, r_2, r_{2L}, do not affect the objective functions.

8 Concluding Remarks

Optimization of the design of the landing slope was carried out. The developed procedure for optimizing the design of the landing slope would be applicable not only to Zao in Yamagata city, but also to all ski jumping hills in the world. The content of the paper is summarized as follows:

- Four objective functions, namely the construction cost, the landing velocity, the flight distance and the standard deviation in the flight distance due to the jumpers' skill differences, were considered.
- It is possible to control the four objective functions by changing the profile of the landing slope.
- Safety on landing (the landing velocity) is almost equivalent to the standard deviation in the flight distance due to differences in the jumpers' skill.
- There is a trade-off between long flight distance and safety on landing and the standard deviation in the flight distance due to differences in the jumpers' skill.
- The construction cost is influenced by the horizontal distance between the edge of the take-off table and the K-point.
- The safety on landing, the flight distance and the standard deviation in the flight distance due to differences in the jumpers' skill are influenced by the ratio of the height difference and the horizontal distance between the edge of the take-off table and the K-point.

Acknowledgements. This work is supported by a Grant-in-Aid for Scientific Research (A), No. 15H01824, Japan Society for the Promotion of Science.

References

1. Seo, K., Watanabe, I., Murakami, M.: Aerodynamic force data for a V-style ski jumping flight. Sports Eng. **7**, 31–39 (2004)
2. McNeil, A.J., Hubbard, M., Swedberg, A.D.: Designing tomorrow's snow park jump. Sports Eng. **15**, 1–20 (2012)
3. Kobayakawa, M., Kondo, Y.: The flight mechanics of ski jumping (in Japanese). Science (Japanese edition) **55–3**, 185–190 (1985)
4. Gasser, H.: Standards for the construction of jumping hills - 2012, Application to Rule 411 of ICR, vol. 3, FIS (International Ski Federation) (2012)
5. Seo, K., Kobayashi, O., Murakami, M.: Multi-optimisation of the screw kick in rugby by using a genetic algorithm. Sports Eng. **9**, 87–96 (2006)
6. Kohonen, T.: Self-organizing Maps. Springer, Heidelberg (1995)

Computer Supported Analysis of Thermal Comfort for Cycling Sport

Alessandro Pezzoli[1(✉)] and Roberto Bellasio[2]

[1] Interuniversity Department of Regional and Urban Studies and Planning,
Politecnico di Torino and Università di Torino, Torino, Italy
alessandro.pezzoli@polito.it
[2] Enviroware, Concorezzo, Italy
rbellasio@enviroware.com

Abstract. This research presents an innovative methodology to evaluate the thermal comfort of cycling athletes. It is well known that the thermal comfort of the athletes is linked with their sport performance and safety. The paper describes a computer supported analysis performed for the two venues of the cycling sport (Time Trial and Road Race) of the 2016 Olympic Games in Rio de Janeiro (Brazil). The meteorological data of two stations representative of the racing areas have been collected for a period of 20 years. They have been analyzed to produce the wind roses, the average typical days of the meteorological variables, and to calculate two important thermal indices: Predicted Mean Vote (PMV) and Physiological Equivalent Temperature (PET). The results of this research show the importance of the climatological analysis for optimizing the training and nutrition plans of the athletes.

Keywords: Thermal comfort · Weather · Computer analysis · Cycling · Sport performance

1 Introduction

As shown in a previous paper [1], the assessment of bio-climatological conditions and of thermal comfort in endurance sports, particularly in road cycling, is essential not only for a proper planning of the training program and the nutritional plan, but also for a better evaluation of the racing strategy or for the correct development and choice of the materials.

Among the meteorological variables that strongly influence the sport activity the most important ones are temperature, wind, precipitation, fog, atmospheric pressure and relative humidity.

In fact Brocherie et al. [2] suggest how an integration of the combination of all relevant multidisciplinary data (i.e. thermal physiology, mathematical modelling, occupational medicine, biometeorology) would generate better application in an eco-logical sport science setting with potential impact on heat stress guideline management.

A deeper review about the emerging environmental and weather challenges in outdoor sports was held by Brocherie et al. [3]. The Authors show how the Universal Thermal Climate Index, also indicated by the abbreviation UTCI [4] promises to be, in the next future, useful for the sport practitioners [5, 6].

© Springer International Publishing AG 2016
J. Cabri and P. Pezarat Correia (Eds.): icSPORTS 2015, CCIS 632, pp. 71–85, 2016.
DOI: 10.1007/978-3-319-52770-3_6

In fact the operational UTCI procedure, classified into ten categories of thermal stress ranging from "extreme cold stress" to "extreme heat stress" [7], appears useful. It promises to assess the outdoor sport participants' physiological responses to humidity and radiative loads in hot environments, as well as to wind in the cold.

Nevertheless Blazejczyk et al. [8] illustrated how, in a comparison between UTCI and other bioclimatic indices, values most similar to those of UTCI were found for indices derived from human heat balance models as Physiological Equivalent Temperature (PET). Similarly to the UTCI, PET also is related to the equivalent temperature. The differences between the specific values of these two indeces result from the various structures of heat balance models and different definitions of reference conditions.

However Pezzoli et al. [9] and Brocherie and Millet [10] show how also the Predicted Mean Vote (PMV) can be used to characterize the thermal comfort in sport activities (respectively for cycling and tennis).

As shown by Brocherie and Millet [10] the WBGT is indicated by numerous leading sports federations (e.g., Fédération Internationale de Football Association [FIFA], International Association of Athletics Federations [IAAF], International Tennis Federation [ITF]) as the index to be used to evaluate the thermal comfort during the sports activities. It is important to remember that this empirical index is computed from the reading of the dry-bulb temperature and two derived measures: the natural wet-bulb temperature and the black-globe temperature.

Moreover the same Authors, based on previous researches, denoted that incorporating newly available bioclimatic indices such as PMV instead of WBGT would considerably improve sport-specific heat stress modeling and current guidelines.

The main goal of this paper is to present an innovative methodology to evaluate the thermal comfort of the athletes considering PET and PMV indices for cycling sport. The analysis will be carried out for the Rio de Janeiro area considering the two venues for the cycling sport and for the two disciplines (Time Trial and Road Race).

This analysis will be developed considering the men's races. The developed statistical analysis will demonstrate how it is possible to characterize the thermal conditions of an athlete involved in a race. Finally this analysis can be used to develop the strategy's assessment of the race.

2 Materials and Methods

2.1 Research Design

The research is developed analyzing:

- The geographical data of the race area with a particular focus on the tracks. For this analysis Google Earth is used as Open Access map system, as well as the free information available on Internet.
- The meteorological data (wind direction, wind speed, air temperature, relative humidity, cloud coverage). This computer supported analysis has been performed using the WindRose PRO3 software. For detailed information about this software, please access: (http://www.enviroware.com/portfolio/windrose-pro3/).

- The PET and the PMV thermal comfort indices. This part of research is also computer-supported through the RayMan software [11, 12].

2.2 Material

Geographical Data. To analyze the geographical data, the first step is searching the tracks that will be used for the two disciplines (Time Trial and Road Race) during Rio de Janeiro 2016 Olympic Games.

This information is provided by Union Cycliste International – International Cycling Union (http://www.uci.ch/road/ucievents/2016-road-olympic-games/196852016/). In the UCI web-page it is possible to find the tracks for the two disciplines.

Then the tracks are georeferenced using Google Earth as Open Access map system (Fig. 1).

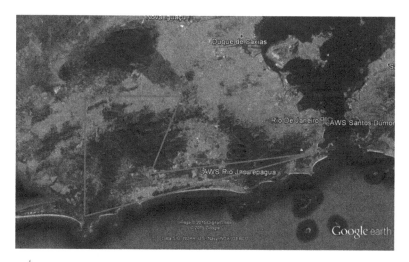

Fig. 1. Positions of the two meteorological stations. In the red box the zone of competence for the road races is indicated. (Color figure online)

Meteorological Data. The meteorological variables, needed for the analysis described in this study, are wind direction, wind speed, air temperature and relative humidity. The meteorological observations at surface have been obtained from the Jacarepagua and Santos Dumont weather stations, whose locations are shown in Fig. 1. The distance between the two stations is about 22 km.

Weather data have been collected for the time period 1994–2014 (20 years). The meteorological data have been analysed filtering out all the values that were not measured in August, because the Olympic Games will be held in Rio de Janeiro between 5th and 21st August 2016.

The WindRose PRO3 Software. A wind rose is a chart which gives a view of how wind speed and wind direction are distributed at a particular location over a specific period of time. This representation allows summarizing in a single plot a large quantity of data; therefore it is a very useful tool.

The wind roses presented in this work have been produced with the WindRose PRO3 software (http://www.enviroware.com/portfolio/windrose-pro3/).

A time filter option allows analysing the wind data and produce wind roses only for particular years, months, days of the week or hours of the day. It is also possible to produce wind roses only for day or night hours, which are determined by the software itself starting from the geographical position and the time zone of the meteorological station. Monthly, hourly and three-hourly wind roses are automatically created by the software.

Also the analysis of the typical day can be carried-out. The typical day is a chronological graph representing the average hourly value of an assigned meteorological variable (i.e.: wind direction, wind speed, air temperature, etc....) along the day.

The WindRose PRO3 software has been used in many sectors: meteorology, architecture, air quality, oceanography, veterinary medicine, veterinary epidemiology, wind energy, climate, aquatic botany and agriculture. It has also been used for the analysis of sport performances [13, 14].

The RayMan Software. The RayMan software [11, 12] is widely employed in bioclimatological studies applied to tourism activities and sport practices. Such software combines many heat transfer models with the heat sensation perceived in the human body. It generates universal scales of thermal sensation, which have large application in the outdoor sports like road cycling [9, 15, 16]. The input variables needed by the RayMan software are:

- Date, hour and location (longitude and latitude, altitude and time zone).
- Environmental and meteorological data like air temperature (°C), pressure (hPa), relative humidity (%), wind speed (m/s) and cloud covering (octas).
- Personal data about the subject (weight, height, age and sex).
- The heat transfer resistance of the clothing, according with UNI EN ISO 9920/2004 and the internal heat production (W), consequential to the physical activity of the subject.

The outputs of the model are the two bioclimatological indices (PMV and PET) which provide the thermal perception and the grade of physiological stress, as reported in Table 1.

The PMV predicts the normalized value of the thermal comfort of a large group of people exposed to similar environmental conditions, while the PET has detailed thermo-physiological basis taking into account the energy balance of the human body in relationship with climatic conditions.

Table 1. Thermal sensations according to PMV and PET values.

PMV	PET [°C]	Thermal perception	Grade of physiological stress
<−3.5	<4	Very cold	Extreme cold stress
−3.5 ÷ −2.5	4 ÷ 8	Cold	Strong cold stress
−2.5 ÷ −1.5	8 ÷ 13	Cool	Moderate cold stress
−1.5 ÷ −0.5	13 ÷ 18	Slightly cool	Slight cold stress
−0.5 ÷ 0.5	18 ÷ 23	Comfortable	No thermal stress
0.5 ÷ 1.5	23 ÷ 29	Slightly warm	Slight heat stress
1.5 ÷ 2.5	29 ÷ 35	Warm	Moderate heat stress
2.5 ÷ 3.5	35 ÷ 41	Hot	Strong heat stress
>3.5	>41	Very hot	Extreme heat stress

2.3 Methods

The Evaluation of Meteorological Conditions for Cycling Sport. As well described by Pezzoli et al. [9] the cycling sport is strongly influenced by the meteorological variables. The wind direction, as well as the wind speed, strongly influences the performance in the cycling sport.

A correct climatological analysis, taking into account this meteorological variable (wind), can be fruitfully used by the coaches and the athletes to:

- Decide the training program (physical and mental);
- Decide about the training site;
- Decide about the nutrition planning;
- Develop the material.

For what concerns the analysis of the wind direction, it is decided to analyse the "True Wind Direction" (TWD) failing to take into account the apparent wind generated by the speed of the bicycle. The TWD is measured in degrees considering the Geographical North. The wind roses (Sect. 3.2) are drawn considering a wind direction range of 30°.

Of course it is evident that also the air temperature and the relative humidity influence the performance in the cycling sport. In fact, as mentioned before, the thermal comfort indices are function of these two meteorological variables.

The typical day of each meteorological variable has been evaluated by using the WindRose PRO3 software. The hourly average wind direction, hourly average wind speed, hourly average air temperature and hourly average relative humidity as well as the hourly standard deviation for all of these meteorological variables are calculated in the typical day.

Finally the rain, evaluated in term of cloud coverage, is analysed and used as input in the RayMan model for the evaluation of the PET and PMV thermal indices.

The Evaluation of Thermal Comfort Conditions for Cycling Sport. The analysis of the thermal comfort was carried out considering the men's category.

The thermal comfort indices (PET and PMV) are evaluated for a target of athletes that represents an average professional "climbing and trialist" cyclist's categories (age: 27, height: 1,75 m, weight: 65 kg as suggested by Lucia et al. [17]).

It was decided to calculate the thermal comfort indices for each hour for a time interval included between 09.00LT ÷ 16.00LT. The input, for what concerns the meteorological variables, are the average of the meteorological variables corrected using the standard deviation.

Moreover the indices are calculated for two different conditions: restore and effort period. The internal heat production (W) is considered equal to 80 W for the restore period and equal to 300 W for the effort period [9].

The heat transfer resistance of the clothing is considered equal to 0.6clo (corresponding to a light gym suit with a t-shirt) for the restore period and equal to 0.3clo (corresponding to a t-shirt and short pants) for the effort period.

3   Results and Discussion

3.1   Analysis of the Venues for Cycling Sports in Rio de Janeiro 2016 Olympic Games

The venues for cycling sports are localized in two areas of Rio de Janeiro named Barra (Time Trial) and Copacabana (Road Race) as illustrated in Fig. 2.

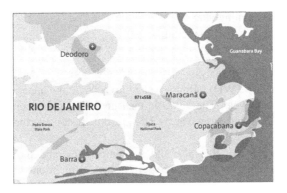

Fig. 2. Location of the two areas for cycling sports in Rio de Janeiro (courtesy: Rio 2016 Organising Committee, http://www.rio2016.com/mapa-de-instalacoes).

A more detailed geographical representation of the two different circuits is provided by UCI. Figure 3 illustrates the circuit of the Time Trial, for a total length of 54.5 km, while Fig. 4 represents the circuit of the Road Race, for a total length of 241.5 km.

Comparing Figs. 3 and 4 with Fig. 1 it is possible to observe that the selected weather stations are representative of both the circuits. Specifically the weather station of Santos Dumont is the reference for Copacabana area and the weather station of Jacarepagua is representative for Barra area.

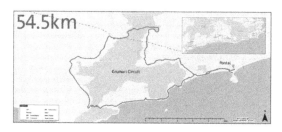

Fig. 3. Time Trial circuit (courtesy: UCI, http://www.uci.ch/road/ucievents/2016-road-olympic-games/196852016/).

It is also evident how the Time Trial race will be carried out in Barra region, while the Road Race will be held both in Copacabana (start and arrival) and in Barra region.

3.2 Analysis of Meteorological Conditions in Rio de Janeiro in August

The wind roses are shown in Figs. 5a, b, c, d and 6a, b, c, d, respectively for the stations Jacarepagua and Santos Dumont. For each station the wind roses have been produced for the period 5–21 August and for four time intervals of the day: 09.00LT ÷ 11.00LT, 12.00LT ÷ 14.00LT, 15.00LT ÷ 17.00LT and 18.00LT ÷ 20.00LT.

At the Jacarepagua station the prevailing wind comes from the north eastern sector in the time interval 09.00LT ÷ 11.00LT, from the southern sector in the time periods 12.00LT ÷ 14.00LT and 15.00LT ÷ 17.00LT, and from the south western sector in the time interval 18.00LT ÷ 20.00LT. In all the time intervals wind speed from 1 m/s to 3 m/s interests about 40% of the observations, while wind speed greater than 5 m/s interests about 5% ÷ 7% of the observations, with the exception of the time period 18.00LT ÷ 20.00LT where it is 2.3%. This last time interval is also characterized by a high value of calms (43%).

At the Santos Dumont station the prevailing wind comes from the northern sector in the time interval 09.00LT ÷ 11.00LT, and from the southern sector in the remaining time intervals.

In the first time interval wind speeds from 1 m/s to 3 m/s interest about 44% of the observations, in the second and fourth time intervals they interest about 25% of the observations, while in the third time interval they interest about the 10% of the observations. The third time interval is also characterized by the higher percentage of wind speeds greater than 5 m/s (more than 30%) and by the lower presence of calms (3.5%).

Considering the positions of the weather stations (Fig. 1), the pattern described by the wind roses is typical of the breeze regimes, with wind blowing from land to sea in the first hours of the morning, and in the opposite direction during the afternoon.

It is possible to note from Fig. 7 as, in the typical day for the Jacarepagua station in August, the wind speed increases in the early afternoon associated to the shift in the South of the wind direction.

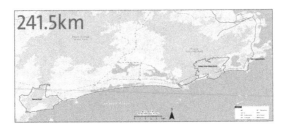

Fig. 4. Road Race circuit (courtesy: UCI, http://www.uci.ch/road/ucievents/2016-road-olympic-games/196852016/).

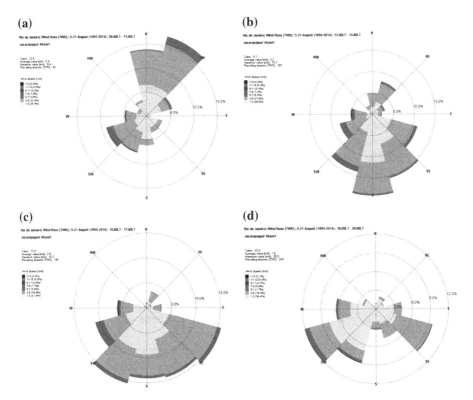

Fig. 5. a. Wind roses of the Jacarepagua station. Time interval: 09.00LT ÷ 11.00LT. **b.** Wind roses of the Jacarepagua station. Time interval: 12.00LT ÷ 14.00LT. **c.** Wind roses of the Jacarepagua station. Time interval: 15.00LT ÷ 17.00LT. **d.** Wind roses of the Jacarepagua station. Time interval: 18.00LT ÷ 20.00LT.

In the same time, from Fig. 8, it is possible to note as, in the same station (Jacarepagua) and in the early afternoon, the air temperature increases and the air humidity decreases.

The decreasing of the air humidity, also if it is associated to an increasing of the air temperature, generates, generally, a false idea that the thermal comfort improves.

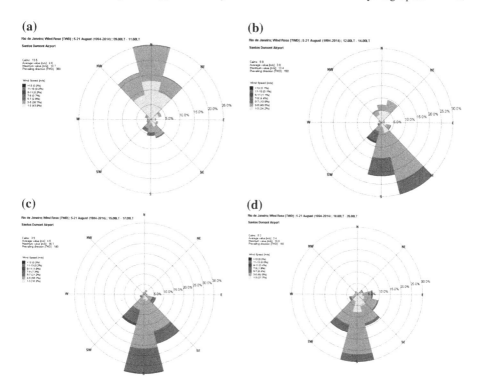

Fig. 6. a. Wind roses of the Santos Dumont station. Time interval: 09.00LT ÷ 11.00LT. **b.** Wind roses of the Santos Dumont station. Time interval: 12.00LT ÷ 14.00LT. **c.** Wind roses of the Santos Dumont station. Time interval: 15.00LT ÷ 17.00LT. **d.** Wind roses of the Santos Dumont station. Time interval: 18.00LT ÷ 20.00LT.

Instead, as it will be shown in the Sect. 3.3, this atmospheric situation will generate a deterioration of the thermal comfort.

This atmospheric pattern is confirmed also in the Santos Dumont (area of Copacabana). In fact from Fig. 9 it is possible to observe the increasing of the wind speed in the afternoon associated to the shift of the wind direction in the South. In the same hours there is a decreasing of the relative air humidity and an increasing of the air temperature (Fig. 10).

3.3 Analysis of Thermal Comfort in Rio de Janeiro in August for the Athletes of Cycling Sports

To analyze the thermal comfort in Rio de Janeiro the two tables, presented by Blazejczyk et al. [8] and Brocherie and Millet [10], are the reference. These tables show the heat-stress indices' temperature limits in reference to thermal sensation, alert description and recommended sporting activity.

Table 2 summarizes the above mentioned tables.

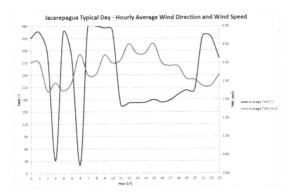

Fig. 7. Jacarepagua typical day: hourly average wind direction and wind speed.

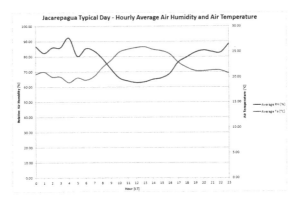

Fig. 8. Jacarepagua typical day: hourly average air humidity and air temperature.

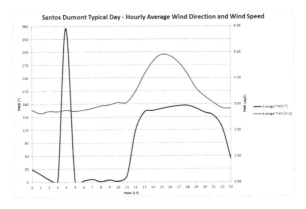

Fig. 9. Santos Dumont typical day: hourly average wind direction and wind speed.

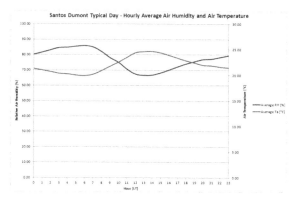

Fig. 10. Santos Dumont typical day: hourly average air humidity and air temperature.

Table 2. Selected heat—stress indices', temperature limits [°C] in reference to thermal sensations, alert description and recommended sporting activity. Modification of the tables of Blazejczyk et al. [8] and of Brocherie and Millet [10].

Thermal sensation	Alert description[a]	Reccomended sporting activity[a]	Index			
			WBGT [°C]	PET [°C]	PMV	UTCI [°C]
Neutral	Generally safe	Unlimited/normal activity	<18	18 ÷ 23	−0.5 ÷ 0.5	9 ÷ 26
Warm	Caution	Increase exercise-to-rest ratio. Decrease intensity and total duration of activity	18 ÷ 24[d]	23 ÷ 35	0.5 ÷ 2.5	26 ÷ 32
Hot	Extreme caution	Activity of unfit, unacclimatized, high-risk[b,c] subjects should be curtailed	24 ÷ 28	35 ÷ 41	2.5 ÷ 3.5	32 ÷ 38
Very hot	Danger	Activity for all except well acclimatized should be stopped	28 ÷ 30	>41	>3.5	38 ÷ 46
Sweltering	Extreme danger	Cancel or stop all practice and competition	>30[e]			>46

[a] Alert description/recommended sport activity for WBGT.
[b] While wearing shorts, t-shirt, ankle socks and sneakers.
[c] Internal heat production exceeds heat loss and core body temperature rises continuously without a plateau.
[d] Threshold (WBGT = 21°C) recommended by marathon organization in northern latitutdes.
[e] Threshold (WBGT > 30°C) recommended by most sporting governing bodies (i.e.: American College of Sport Medicine [ACSM], International Tennis Federation [ITF], Women's Tennis Association [WTA] and Fédération Internationale de Football Association [FIFA]).

Figures 11 and 12 illustrate the PET and PMV in the restore period for Copacabana and Barra areas (Sect. 2.3).

Observing Figs. 11 and 12, it is possible to note that around 12.00LT the thermal indices reach high values (PET = 27 ÷ 31°C; PMV = 1.1 ÷ 1.7) for both the areas. It is also important to note that in Copacabana the values of the thermal comfort indices are lower than those obtained in the Barra area.

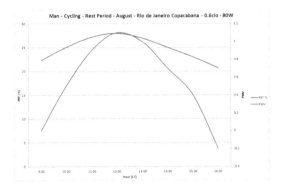

Fig. 11. PET and PMV thermal indices in the restore period for Rio de Janeiro Copacabana area.

The maximum values of PET and PMV observed in Figs. 11 and 12 correspond to a warm thermal sensation and an alert description, as recommended for sporting activity for WBGT, equal to "caution".

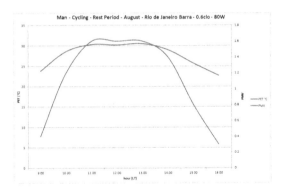

Fig. 12. PET and PMV thermal indices in the restore period for Rio de Janeiro Barra area.

In the early morning, as well as in the afternoon, the indices show a comfortable situation from a thermal comfort point of view.

The values obtained in this analysis show that, in the restore period, the clothing suites are to be changed during the day moving from light gym suit with a t-shirt to t-shirt and short pants.

Finally, the PET and the PMV values in the effort period for Copacabana and Barra areas (Sect. 2.3) are shown in Figs. 13 and 14.

Also for the effort period, the maximum values of the PET and the PMV are confirmed between 12.00LT ÷ 13.00LT (PET = 27 ÷ 30°C; PMV = 3.2 ÷ 3.7).

It is possible to note as the PET values during the effort period are similar to the PET values during the restore period. These results are function of a correct choice of clothing that the athletes have to use during the race and the restore period (Sect. 2.3).

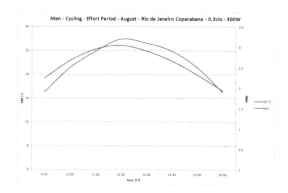

Fig. 13. PET and PMV thermal indices in the effort period for Rio de Janeiro Copacabana area.

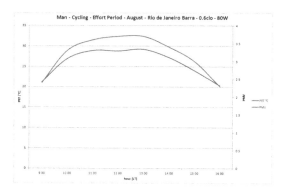

Fig. 14. PET and PMV thermal indices in the effort period for Rio de Janeiro Barra area.

However the PMV values in the effort period are higher than the PMV values of the restore period. Generally it is possible to observe as the maximum values of the PET and PMV indices correspond to a "caution – extreme caution" alert description recommended for sporting activity for WBGT.

The same recommendations show that, in these conditions, it is important to increase the exercise-to-rest ratio as well as to decrease the intensity and the total duration of activity. In the same time it is very important that the athletes are well acclimatized and that they prepare a correct plan and strategy for nutrition and hydration (pre-event, event, post-event).

4   Conclusions

The analysis of the thermal comfort of the athletes during the next Rio de Janeiro Olympic Games, made with an innovative methodology, is presented in this research. The calculations have been carried out for the men's category of the cycling sport. The meteorological data of a 20-year long period have been collected for two monitoring stations that are representative for the race areas (Time Trial and Road Race). The data of the months of August have been analyzed in order to create the wind roses and the typical days of the main variables. Two thermal comfort indices (PET and PMV) have then been calculated considering also the clothing type and the power generated during the exercise. They have been determined for the time period 09.00LT $\div$ 16.00LT and for the resting and effort phases of both races.

It is important to note how the presented methodology can be generalized to other sport as well as to other venues. In fact the presented RayMan model takes into account the personal data about the subject (weight, height, age and sex) as well as the internal heat production (W) consequential to her/his physical activity.

Then it will be possible to change these reference data to adapt the methodology and the model to the analysed sport.

Finally, in the future, it will be interesting to quantify the thermal comfort of the athletes measuring directly the skin's temperature and the skin's humidity of the athletes [9]. This innovation in the research will help to quantify correctly the thermal comfort and to improve the alert description and the recommended sporting activity (Table 2).

For these reasons, the procedure described in this study gives useful information about the most suitable clothing type for affording the race. The results are also useful for defining pre, during and post-race nutrition and hydration plans.

References

1. Pezzoli, A., Cristofori, E., Moncalero, M., Giacometto, F., Boscolo, A., Bellasio, R., Padoan, J.: Effect of the environment on the sport performance: computer supported training – a case study for the cycling sports. In: Cabri, J., Pezarat Correia, P., Barreiros, J. (eds.) Sport Science Research and Technology Support, pp. 1–16. Springer, London (2015)
2. Brocherie, F., Girard, O., Pezzoli, A., Millet, G.P.: Outdoor exercise performance in ambient heat: time to overcome challenging factors? Int. J. Hyperth. **30**(8), 547–549 (2014)
3. Brocherie, F., Girard, O., Millet, G.P.: Emerging environmental and weather challenges in outdoor sports. In: Pezzoli, A. (ed.) Climate – Special Issue "Climate Impacts on Health", vol. 3, pp. 492–521. MDPI, Basel (2015)
4. Jendritzky, G., Maarouf, G., Fiala, D., Staiger, H.: An up-date on the development of a universal thermal climate index. In: Proceedings of the 15th Conference on Biometeorology/Aerobiology and 16th International Congress of Biometeorology, pp. 129–133. AMS, Kansas City (2002)
5. Bröde, P., Błazejczyk, K., Fiala, D., Havenith, G., Holmér, I., Jendritzky, G., Kuklane, K., Kampmann, B.: The Universal Thermal Climate Index UTCI compared to ergonomics standards for assessing the thermal environment. Ind. Health **51**, 16–24 (2013)
6. Pappenberger, F., Jendritzky, G., Staiger, H., Dutra, E., Di Giuseppe, F., Richardson, D.S., Cloke, H.L.: Global forecasting of thermal health hazards: the skill of probabilistic predictions of the Universal Thermal Climate Index (UTCI). Int. J. Biometeorol. **59**, 311–323 (2015)

7. Brode, P., Fiala, D., Blazejczyk, K., Holmer, I., Jendritzky, G., Kampmann, B., Tinz, B., Havenith, G.: Deriving the operational procedure for the Universal Thermal Climate Index (UTCI). Int. J. Biometeorol. **56**, 481–494 (2012)
8. Blazejczyk, K., Epstein, Y., Jendritzky, G., Staiger, H., Tinz, B.: Comparison of UTCI to selected thermal indices. Int. J. Biometeorol. **56**, 515–535 (2012)
9. Pezzoli, A., Cristofori, E., Gozzini, B., Marchisio, M., Padoan, J.: Analysis of the thermal comfort in cycling athletes. Procedia Eng. **34**, 433–438 (2012)
10. Brocherie, F., Millet, G.P.: Is the Wet-Bulbe Globe Temperature (WBGT) Index relevant for exercise in the heat? Sports Med. (2015). doi:10.1007/s40279-015-0386-8
11. Matzarakis, A., Rutz, F., Mayer, H.: Modelling Radiation fluxes in simple and complex environments – Application of the RayMan model. Int. J. Biometeorol. **51**, 323–334 (2007)
12. Matzarakis, A., Rutz, F., Mayer, H.: Modelling Radiation fluxes in simple and complex environments: basics of the RayMan model. Int. J. Biometeorol. **54**, 131–139 (2010)
13. Pezzoli, A., Baldacci, A., Cama, A., Faina, M., Dalla Vedova, D., Besi, M., Vercelli, G., Boscolo, A., Moncalero, M., Cristofori, E., Dalessandro, M.: Wind-wave interactions in enclosed basins: the impact on the sport of rowing. In: Clanet, C. (ed.) Sport Physics, pp. 139–151. Ecole Polytechnique de Paris, Paris (2013)
14. Pezzoli, A., Bellasio, R.: Analysis of wind data for sports performance design: a case study for sailing sports. Sports **2**(4), 99–130 (2014)
15. Matzarakis, A., Mayer, H., Iziomon, M.G.: Application of a universal thermal index: physiological equivalent temperature. Int. J. Biometeorol. **43**, 76–84 (1999)
16. Brandenburg, C., Matzarakis, A., Arnberger, A.: Weather and cycling – a first approach to the effects of weather conditions on cycling. Meteorol. Appl. **14**, 61–67 (2007)
17. Lucia, A., Joyos, H., Chicarro, J.L.: Physiological response to professional road cycling: climber vs. time trialist. Int. J. Sports Med. **21–7**, 505–512 (2000)

Met-Ocean and Heeling Analysis During the Violent 21/22 October 2014 Storm Faced by the Sailboat ECO40 in the Gulf of Lion: Comparison Between Measured and Numerical Wind Data

Paolo De Girolamo[1], Alessandro Romano[1(✉)], Giorgio Bellotti[2],
Alessandro Pezzoli[3], Myrta Castellino[1], Mattia Crespi[1], Augusto Mazzoni[1],
Marcello Di Risio[4], Davide Pasquali[4], Leopoldo Franco[2], and Paolo Sammarco[5]

[1] DICEA, Sapienza Università di Roma, Via Eudossiana, 18, 00184 Roma, Italy
{paolo.degirolamo,alessandro.romano,
mattia.crespi,augusto.mazzoni}@uniroma1.it
[2] Dip. di Ingegneria, Università di Roma Tre,
Via Vito Volterra, 62, 00146 Roma, Italy
{giorgio.bellotti,leopoldo.franco}@uniroma3.it
[3] DIST, L.R. MeteoSport, Politecnico di Torino and Università di Torino,
Viale Mattioli 39, 10125 Torino, Italy
alessandro.pezzoli@polito.it
[4] DICEAA, Laboratorio di Idraulica Ambientale e Marittima LIAM,
Università dellAquila, P.le Pontieri, 1, 67040 Monteluco di Roio, LAquila, Italy
{marcello.dirisio,davide.pasquali}@univaq.it
[5] DICII, Università di Roma Tor Vergata, Via del Politecnico, 1, 00133 Roma, Italy
sammarco@ing.uniroma2.it

Abstract. On 19 October 2014 Matteo Miceli, a known italian oceanic sailor, left the Port of Riva di Traiano (Rome, IT) with the italian sailing boat ECO 40, for the Roma Ocean World Project. This ambitious challenge consists of a non-stop sailing alone around the World in energy and food self-sufficiency. ECO 40 is a Class 40 oceanic vessel (LOA of 12,0 m) that has been equipped with a data acquisition system for measuring both the met-ocean parameters recorded (apparent and real wind speed and wind direction, atmospheric pressure, current velocity, air temperature, sea temperature, etc.) and the kinematic characteristics of the boat itself (i.e., speed and course over ground). Furthermore, the boat has been equipped with three high precision GPS receivers, provided by Leica Geosystem, for measuring the motion of the boat and an inertial platform. Due to these high-precision instruments it is possible to fully measure and characterize the six degrees of freedom of the boat, and accordingly to use her as a sailing wave buoy. Within this paper we present the analysis of the met-ocean data measured by the boat during the storm occurred in the Gulf of Lion on the 21–22 October 2014 that ECO 40 has faced just few days after her departure. Furthermore, by analyzing the GPS signals by means of an innovative application of differential kinematic positioning technique, a detailed analysis of the boat

© Springer International Publishing AG 2016
J. Cabri and P. Pezarat Correia (Eds.): icSPORTS 2015, CCIS 632, pp. 86–105, 2016.
DOI: 10.1007/978-3-319-52770-3_7

heeling during the Gulf of Lion event has been carried out. The boat heeling measurements have been used to correct the measured wind data that have been compared with the hindcast time series.

Keywords: Sailing boat · Waves · Wind · Forecast

1 Introduction and Aim of the Research

On October 19, 2014 Matteo Miceli, a famous Italian oceanic sailor, left the Port of Riva di Traiano located close to Rome (Italy) with the Italian sailboat ECO40 for the Roma Ocean World Project. This ambitious challenge consists in a non-stop sailing alone around the World in energy and food self-sufficiency. The planned route was the classic clipper route which runs from West to East through the Southern Ocean, to take advantage of the strong westerly winds. Namely the route, very similar to that of several prominent yacht races as Around Alone and Vende Globe, consists in passing the Gibraltar Strait, then in descending the Atlantic Ocean and sailing around the Antarctic, at an average latitude of 50S, from west to east rounding the most famous capes of the world: Cape of Good Hope, Cape Leeuwin and Cape Horn. Finally, sailing the Atlantic Ocean back to the Strait of Gibraltar coming back to the homeport. The total distance to be covered by the sailboat was estimated in about 28,000 nautical miles, while the duration was estimated in about five months.

When Matteo was on the way back to Italy, after rounding the three capes and sailing for 25.000 nautical miles, ECO40 capsized at the equator. He was about 600 miles offshore the Brazilian coasts. Matteo was saved by a cargo. When he came back to Italy, he organized a first expedition with four friends to try to recover ECO40, which was not successful. After one month they tried again and found ECO40 300 miles offshore the Brazilian coasts. Now ECO40 is back in Italy.

ECO40 is a Class 40 oceanic vessel (LOA of 12,0 m) that has been equipped with a data acquisition system for both the met-ocean parameters recorded on-board (i.e. apparent and real wind speed and wind direction, atmospheric pressure, current velocity, air and sea temperature, etc.) and the kinematic characteristics of the boat itself (i.e. speed and course over ground). Furthermore, the boat has been equipped with a three high precision GPS receivers, provided by Leica Geosystem, for measuring the movements of the boat and with an inertial platform. Thanks to these instruments it is possible to fully measure and characterize the six degrees of freedom of the boat.

In order to reduce the significant cost of the data transfer by satellite modem just a small part of the measured data was sent to the land team on daily basis. The sampling frequency for the met-ocean data acquisition is 2 Hz, nevertheless only the data averaged over a time window of 10 min were sent to shore. These data, measured by the boat and transmitted almost in real time, helped significantly the team in charge of the safety of ECO40; in fact the knowledge of the actual weather conditions that the boat is really facing during her navigation can improve the route strategy and increase the boat safety. Furthermore, the boat performance data (i.e. speed and course over ground) can allow, after a certain amount of time that is required to obtain a statistically meaningful database, to estimate the real polar velocity curves of the boat. Indeed these curves were used for the prediction of the optimal route (routage) made by the land team by using a route optimization software, which was sent daily to ECO40.

It is worth noticing that the actual polar velocity curves of the boat differ from the theoretical ones estimated by the designer of the boat. This is due to several causes, among which plays an important role the ability of the crew to "push" the boat to the maximum of its performance and the presence of waves that normally is not taken into account when calculating the curves themselves. The remaining data were supposed to be analyzed once the boat had come back. Fortunately the data were saved together with the boat.

The measurements of the boat movements, obtained from the three GPS receivers, if properly analyzed, can provide a measure of the waves that ECO40 encountered during its navigation. In other words ECO40 can be used as a moving wave buoy for measuring the waves characteristics (i.e. significant wave height H_{m0}, peak period T_p and mean direction θ) experienced during navigation.

These data are used mainly for two technical and scientific purposes. The first purpose is the calibration and/or verification of the numerical models output that are commonly used for the wind and wave forecast and/or analysis into the oceans, and the calibration of the remote sensing data (e.g. satellite wind and wave measurements). The second purpose is directly related to the vessel design. Indeed the knowledge of both the movements and the loads that these kind of vessel can deal with, together with the response of the materials to the fatigue stresses, can improve significantly the design methods.

The aim of this paper consists in analyzing, both in terms of the met-ocean conditions faced by the boat and in terms of the heeling of the boat itself, the first storm experienced by ECO40 during its navigation that occurred in the Gulf of Lion on October 21–22, 2014. The paper is structured as follows. First we present the analysis of the Gulf of Lion weather event. Then the description of the GPS acquisition system, as well as the analysis of the heeling of the boat during the storm itself, are presented and discussed. The description of the available wind and waves data follows. Then we show the results of the comparison between the wind measurements carried out on board and those reconstructed in forecasting and in analysis, by using the numerical data of the GFS (Global Forecast System) and ECMWF (European Center for Medium-range Weather Forecast). Finally, we show a comparison of these storm data with those related to the violent storm that occurred in the Gulf of Lion on 2 November 1995, which caused the sinking of the Italian racing boat Parsifal, killing six of its nine crew members. The weather conditions that caused the sinking of the boat have been reconstructed by [3].

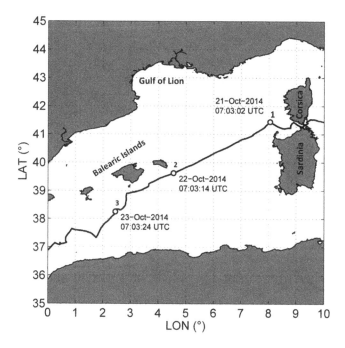

Fig. 1. The route between the Asinara Island and the Balearic Islands that the boat ECO40 has followed.

2 The ECO40's Route During the Gulf of Lion Event

On 19 October 2014, when ECO40 left from the Italian Port Riva di Traiano, the weather conditions appeared to be clear: within the next 24/48 h the first seasonal front of cold air, expected to cause Mistral winds having speed exceeding 40 knots, would come from the Gulf of Lion. Fortunately, ECO40 was able to reach the Asinara Island and began to follow the route towards the Balearic Islands before the arrival of the main storm: the boat has faced the storm running on the quarter. The route between the Asinara Island and the Balearic Islands that the boat ECO40 has followed is represented in Fig. 1. The figure shows also information of the travel times.

Eco 40 has covered about 200 nautical miles in 24 h, with a mean speed of almost 8.3 knots (see points 1 and 2 in Fig. 1). Between the points 1 and 2 (see Fig. 1) ECO40 was fully exposed to the northern quadrants, while on the route between the points 2 and 3 the boat was partially sheltered by the Balearic Islands. Figure 2 shows the plots of the speed over ground (SOG) and of the course over ground (COG) during the Gulf of Lion Event. We recall that these values are averaged over a time interval of 10 min.

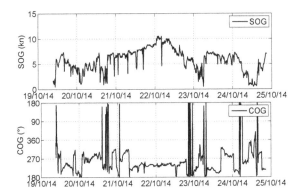

Fig. 2. Time series of the speed over ground (upper panel) and of the course over ground (lower panel) during the Gulf of Lion Event.

3   Weather Analysis of the Gulf of Lion Storm

In the days 20th and 21st October 2014, the atmospheric circulation was characterized by a zonal flux from West to East in the Northern of Europe. A high pressure was centered on the Mediterranean Sea (Fig. 3).

At the same time a frontal system, positioned between a low pressure centered on the Atlantic Ocean and a low pressure centered in the Polands plan, started to move slowly toward South. The movement of this frontal system was generated by the faster change of direction of the zonal flux in the UK island, in turn generated by the movement towards East of the tropical low pressure Gonzalo. The trough in upper atmosphere (see Fig. 4, upper panel) associated with the cold air movement on the day of October 21 and in the night of the October 22 (see Fig. 4, lower panel), generated the movement to South of the cold front (see Fig. 5, upper panel).

When the cold front encountered the Alps, it developed the classical low pressure down-wind to the mountain. Then a low pressure with the center at 998hPa was positioned on the Venice Gulf. The opposition between this low pressure and the high pressure with center at 1033hPa positioned on the Biscay Gulf, jointly with the movement of the cold air in upper atmosphere (see Fig. 5, lower panel), generated an atmospheric situation characterized by an high instability. This weather pattern was active on the Mediterranean Sea for the entire day on October 22, 2014 and for a part of the October 23, 2014 (see Fig. 6).

This particular baric configuration generated strong wind from N on the Mediterranean Sea in particular on the Gulf of Lion, on the West of Mediterranean Sea, on the Sicily Channel and on the Sardinia Channel. Moreover, the slow movement of the cold front and of the low pressure made an adverse meteorological situation for a time as long as 48 h.

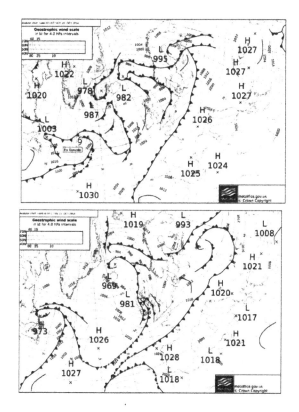

Fig. 3. Upper panel: surface Analysis for 20 October 2014 h 00.00UTC (source: MetOffice). Lower panel: surface Analysis for 21 October 2014 h 00.00UTC (source: MetOffice).

4   Description of the GPS Measurement System

Within this section a brief description of the GPS measurement system is provided. As previously mentioned, three high precision GPS receivers have been installed on the boat. As shown by Fig. 7 two receivers have been placed on the left and right side of the stern along the boat cross axis showed in Fig. 7, while the remaining one has been placed close to the boat entrance along the boat main longitudinal axis (see Fig. 7).

The GPS raw code and phase observations on both L1 and L2 frequencies were acquired by each above described GPS antenna/receiver system with a sampling rate of 2 Hz. The raw observations have been acquired by the system during the navigation of ECO40 and stored on a flash-card by each receiver. The data analysis was carried out in post-processing after the recovery of the flash-cards. Devoted routine has been implemented to read, for each day and for each receiver, the 24 hourly mdb files and to convert them in RINEX (Receiver Independent Exchange Format) daily files. On the basis of this dataset two dif-

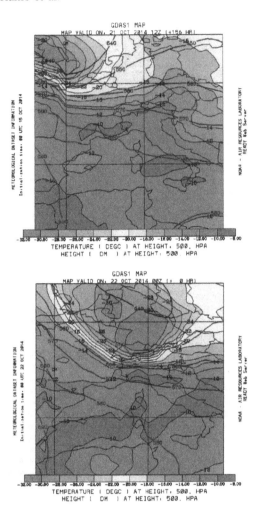

Fig. 4. Upper panel: upper Atmosphere Analysis at 500hPa for 21 October 2014 h 12.00UTC (source: MetOffice). Color filled area: temperature at 500hPa [C]. Red solid line: height level at 500hPa [mx10]. Lower panel: upper Atmosphere Analysis at 500hPa for 22 October 2014 h 00.00UTC (source: MetOffice). Color filled area: temperature at 500hPa [C]. Red solid line: height level at 500hPa [mx10]. (Color figure online)

ferent strategies were adopted in the post-processing: the "Variometric Approach for Displacements Analysis Standalone Engine" (VADASE, [1,2,4–6]) and the moving base kinematic approach.

It is important to highlight that the two methods have been used complementarly in order to obtain the boat motion. Indeed, the first (i.e. variometric approach) has been used to calculate the boat heave motion which is related to wave heights faced by the sailboat, while the second one (i.e. moving base

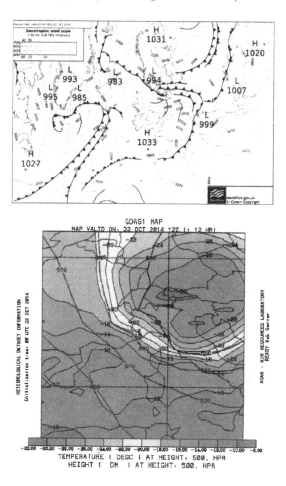

Fig. 5. Upper panel: surface Analysis for 22 October 2014 h 00.00UTC (source: MetOffice). Lower panel: upper Atmosphere Analysis at 500hPa for 22 October 2014 h 12.00UTC (source: MetOffice). Color filled area: temperature at 500hPa [C]. Red solid line: height level at 500hPa [mx10]. (Color figure online)

kinematic approach) has been used to reconstruct the heeling of the sailboat during the off-shore navigation (i.e. far from the coast). Note that wave measurements by means of the GPS signals have not been treated in the present paper, therefore only the latter approach is discussed in the following.

4.1   GPS Data Processing for the Heeling Analysis

Here a brief description of the moving base kinematic technique is provided. The most widely used technique in GPS kinematic positioning is based on double frequency phase observations differential approach (double differences) between the rover moving receiver and a reference static receiver of known coordinates.

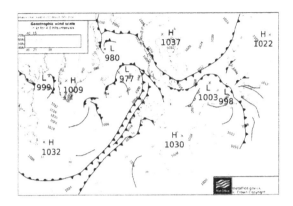

Fig. 6. Surface Analysis for 23 October 2014 h 00.00UTC. (source: MetOffice)

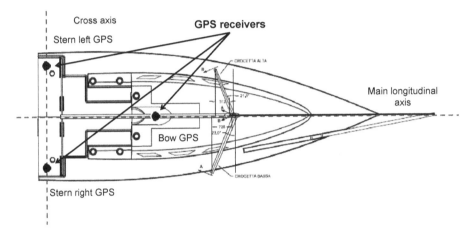

Fig. 7. Sketch of the boat and of the GPS receivers (red dots). (Color figure online)

This technique can be used in real rime (NTRK - Network Real Time Kinematic) or in Post-Processing. It is a highly performing technique (positioning accuracy at few centimeters level), but it requires the support of a reference receiver or a GNSS Network infrastructure. Generally, in order to obtain high accuracy results, the distance between the rover and the reference receiver should not exceede few tens of kilometers, so it is not possible to apply this technique in off-shore navigation case (like the one described within the paper) due to the lack of close reference receivers availability.

Nevertheless, it is possible to apply an unusual approach of the differential kinematic positioning technique to perform a detailed analysis of the boat heeling. It is important to highlight that by applying this technique, and of course by knowing the distance between the receivers, an accurate estimate of their relative positions can be obtained (i.e. for the roll and heeling analysis of the boat) but no information on the absolute positions of the receivers themselves can be obtained.

This approach is briefly described as follows. A reference moving receiver (i.e. stern-right, Fig. 7) has been considered. With respect to this reference moving receiver, it was possible to estimate, epoch by epoch, the positions of the other stern receiver (i.e. stern-left, Fig. 7). In particular, for each acquisition epoch (172800 per day), the position of stern-left receiver was estimated. Daily RINEX from October 20th to October 23rd of the two stern receivers were processed in couple using an open source library [11]; 8 daily solution files (2 per day) were obtained. Each daily solution file (4 for stern-left) contains the epoch-by-epoch positions, of the considered receiver, in terms of East, North ad Up components in a local reference system [7] with origin in stern-right receiver epoch referenced position.

By using the above mentioned technique the heeling angle estimation has been obtained. It is worth noting that for a floating body there are some motions which can be assumed characterized by a zero mean value (e.g. heave and pitch). This allows to avoid bias related to measurements techniques, by using high pass filters. This assumption cannot be used for roll because its mean value, especially for a sailboat, is not zero and coincides with the heeling. Therefore, for the heeling measurement it is very important to use a very precise GPS analysis technique. In this contest the above described method appears to be novel.

By using the signals of the relative vertical positions between the stern-right and the stern-left receivers (i.e. $\Delta z(t)$) between the two receivers in a local reference system), the instantaneous heeling angle α of the boat has been identified. Figure 8 shows the roll and the heeling angles experienced by the boat during the the Gulf of Lion storm. In the figure the black line refers to the instantaneous (2 Hz) values of the roll angle, while the thick red line refers to the averaged values obtained over 10 min which coincides with the heeling. The minimum value of the measured heeling angle ($\alpha \simeq -50°$) occurs during the last few hours of October 22nd when the storm peak is approaching the sailboat. Moreover, Fig. 8 allows to identify the tack changes of the sailboat. It appears that, during the whole storm, the sailboat was mainly on starboard tack.

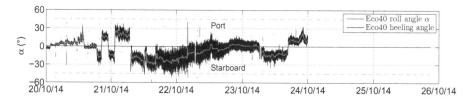

Fig. 8. Measured roll and heeling angles during the Gulf of Lion event. Note: black line refers to the instantaneous values (roll), while the thick red line refers to the averaged values obtained as the mean value of the roll angle α. The red dashed lines refer to the values of the heeling angle $\overline{\alpha} = \pm 45$. (Color figure online)

5 Wind Data Analysis

5.1 Aims of the Analysis

In this section wind data measured on board during the violent Gulf of Lion storm are presented and compared to the numerical data provided in forecasting by the GFS (Global Forecast System) and in analysis by ECMWF (European Center for Medium-range Weather Forecast). The reason for this comparison is dual. The first one concerns the verification of the above mentioned numerical data, while the second one concerns the forecast wind conditions which are provided to a sailing boat for safety reasons, which in the opinion of oceanic sailors are often considered underestimated when severe storms occur. With reference to the introduction of the present paper, wind data measurements used in the following analysis are those transmitted to the shore team by ECO40 almost in real time. These values are:

- the mean apparent and true wind values (speed and direction) computed onboard over a time window of 10 min by using the data acquired at a sampling rate of 2 Hz;
- the maximum value of apparent and true wind speed and direction measured over each 10 min time window (i.e. gusts).

The wind data have been recorded during the whole navigation (about 5 months) by the onboard computer of the boat with a sampling rate of 2 Hz. Nevertheless, after the boat capsizing, the computer remained into the sea water for about 2.5 months. Currently, the work of retrieving data stored by the computer is ongoing. For this reason in the present work only the mean wind and gusts values are used.

5.2 Position of the Anemometer

Wind data have been measured onboard of ECO40 by means of an anemometer placed on the top of the mast at the height $z = +19$ m above the m.s.l., when the boat is in calm water (i.e. no waves) and with a zero roll angle ($\alpha = 0$). This anemometer position (top of the mast) is normally used on sailboats, the anemometer is subjected to a motion. This motion produces two main effects: (i) modify wind measurements (speed and direction); (ii) modify the height of the anemometer. Concerning (i), if boat motion is known, it is possible to determine also the motion of the anemometer in order to depurate instantaneous (2 Hz) wind measurements from it. In the following this aspect has not been taken into consideration because the instantaneous wind measurements, as mentioned, are not still available. It has been only considered the horizontal motion of the boat (surge and sway) in order to calculate the true wind speed and direction from the measured apparent wind. Therefore the attention has been pointed out only to effect (ii). If we want to refer the anemometer height $z(t)$ to the mean sea level, the following approximated relation may be applied (see Fig. 9):

$$z(t) = l \cos \alpha(t) + \eta(t) \tag{1}$$

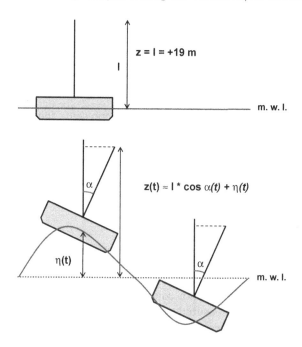

Fig. 9. Sketch of the instantaneous measurement height $z(t)$ as a function of the heeling angle $\alpha(t)$ and of the water free surface elevation $\eta(t)$ referred to the m.w.l.

where l is the mast length, $\alpha(t)$ is the instantaneous roll and $\eta(t)$ is the instantaneous free surface elevation under the boat hull measured with respect to the mean water level. The main approximation of Eq. (1) is due to the term $\eta(t)$. Nevertheless for a light displacement boat such as ECO40, this approximation is in the order of few centimeters. In Eq. (1) the pitch motion of the anemometer has not been included because it is less important than roll and it is characterized by a zero mean value.

Since the wind measurements used in the present work are averaged values over a time window of 10 min, then Eq. (1) has to be averaged in time too. The mean values of Eq. (1) over a time window of 10 min in presence of wind and waves gives:

$$\overline{z(t)} = l \cos \overline{\alpha(t)}, \tag{2}$$

because we can assume that $\eta(t)$ is a zero mean signal and $\overline{\alpha(t)}$ is the heeling angle represented by Fig. 8 (red thick line).

Numerical models provide the wind speed and direction at the conventional height $z = +10$ m above the m.s.l. that is different with respect to the measurement height $\overline{z(t)}$ provided by Eq. (2). Therefore, in order to properly compare the measured speed data with the numerical results, it is necessary to reduce the wind speed to the conventional height $z = +10$m above the m.s.l. This has been carried out by using the vertical profile of the wind speed proposed by [9]. This relationship describes a logarithmic vertical profile of the wind velocity, that has the following functional form:

$$\frac{U_z}{U_{10}} = 1 + \frac{\sqrt{C_{10}} \ln \frac{z}{10}}{C_K} \tag{3}$$

where U_z is the wind speed at the height z, U_{10} represents the wind speed at $z = +10$ m above the mean sea level, C_{10} is a coefficient that is function of the flow regime of the wind speed and of the surface roughness that depends on the wave conditions. In order to estimate C_{10} the functional form proposed by [12] has been used. As shown in the following relationship the coefficient C_{10} depends just on the wind velocity, while it does not take into account directly the wave field

$$C_{10} = 0.65(U_{10})^{1/2} \cdot 10^{-3} \ if \ (U_{10} \leq 15m/s) C_{10} = 0.24 \cdot 10^{-3} \ if \ (U_{10} > 15m/s) \tag{4}$$

C_K represents the Von Karman coefficient, equal to 0.4. Thus, Eq. (3) has been used to evaluate the measured wind speed at the conventional height $z = +10$ m above the mean sea level, once the actual wind speed U_z and the actual measurement height $z = \overline{z(t)}$ are known.

5.3   Wind Measurements Analysis

In this section the direct wind measurements sent to the shore by ECO40 are analized. The true wind speed V_w and the true wind direction θ_w during the Gulf of Lion event, obtained from the apparent wind and from the boat kinematic characteristics computed by the navigation software of the boat, are shown in Fig. 10. The upper panel of Fig. 10 shows the time series of the mean values (i.e. averaged over 10 min) of the true wind speed (black line) and the true wind gust (red line) that represents the highest values of true wind speed measured over 10 min. It is worth noticing that the maximum value of the averaged wind speed reached 45 knots at the peak of the event, while the values of the gusts were greater than 50 knots, reaching a maximum value of 56 knots. The lower panel of Fig. 10 shows the time series of the true wind directions; also in this plot both the quantities that refer to the averaged values and the ones that refer to the gust values are represented. The upper panel of Fig. 11 represents the scatter plot between the averaged true wind speed and the true wind gust.

The plot shows that the wind gust values are generally larger of about 15–20% than the averaged true wind speed; also, the difference between the averaged wind speed and the gusts tends to increase as the wind speed increases. In order to highlight this feature, the functional relationship, as obtained by applying a linear regression to the measured data, has been represented (red line) in the upper panel of Fig. 11.

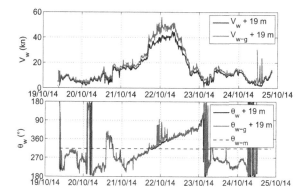

Fig. 10. Upper panel: time series of the true wind speed averaged over 10 min (black line) and of the true wind gust (red line). Lower panel: time series of the true wind direction averaged over 10 min (black line) and of the true wind gust direction (red line); note: the dotted black line refers to the mean direction of the true wind (θ_{w-m} during the event is 313.6). (Color figure online)

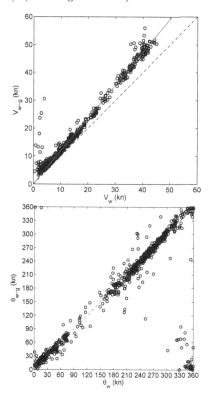

Fig. 11. Upper panel: scatter plot of the averaged true wind speed vs the true wind gust; the red line represents the best line fit, as obtained by applying a linear regression to the measured data. Lower panel: scatter plot of the averaged true wind direction vs the true wind gust direction.

5.4   Comparison of Wind Measurements with Numerical Models Data

In this section the wind measurements are compared with the results provided by the numerical models. This comparison has been carried out into two phases. In the first one, the direct comparison between measurements and numerical models output has been performed, i.e. without modifying the measurement height z of the wind for both the source of data. In some way this represent the oceanic sailor experience who uses the wind forecast in order to prepare the sails trim for the incoming storm and, during the storm, compares the forecasted wind with the actual wind, provided by the anemometer located on the top of the mast. In the second one, the wind speed coming from the two sources is reduced to the same height.

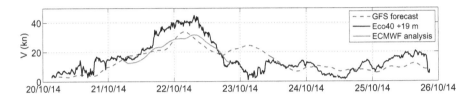

Fig. 12. Direct comparison between the true wind speed (averaged over 10 min) measured at the top of the mast (black line) and the numerical model output of the GFS (dashed red line) and of the ECMWF data in analysis (continuous blue line). (Color figure online)

As previously mentioned, the measured data have been compared with two sources of data. The first comparison has been carried out with the ECMWF (European Centre for Medium-Range Weather Forecasts) analysis data, that are provided with a spatial resolution of 0.125 and with a time resolution of 6 h. A second comparison has been carried out by using the forecast data provided by the numerical model GFS (Global Forecast System). The output of this model, that has a spatial resolution of 1.0 and a time resolution of 3 h, have been used for the routing of ECO40. The comparisons are shown in Fig. 12, that represents the time series of (i) the averaged wind speed (black line) measured by ECO40 by the anemometer placed on the top of the mast (as shown in Fig. 10), and (ii) the time series of the wind speed obtained in analysis and by the GFS, linearly interpolated (in time and space) along the route of the boat between Sardinia Island and the Balearic Islands. The results of the GFS model (i.e. forecast data) are identified by a red dashed line, while the results of the ECMWF model (i.e. analysis data) are identified by a continuous blue line.

The forecast data have been sent to the boat on October 19, 2014, thus it is expected that they have a higher accuracy in the first 24–48 h. Figure 12 shows that the wind speed values measured on board are often larger than those estimated by the numerical models, especially during the peak of the storm. As

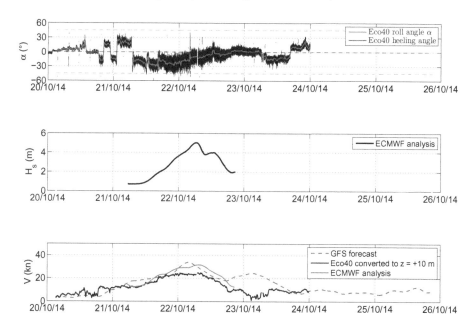

Fig. 13. Upper panel: measured heeling angle $\overline{\alpha}$ during the Gulf of Lion event. Note: black line refers to the instantaneous values (roll), while the thick red line refers to the heeling $\overline{\alpha}$. Middle panel: analysis data (ECMWF) of the significant wave height H_s interpolated (in time and space) along the route of the boat between Sardinia Island and the Balearic Islands. Lower panel: comparison between the true wind speed (averaged over 10 min) evaluated at the height $z = +10$ m above the m.s.l. (black line) obtained by using the Eq. (3) and the numerical model output of the GFS (dashed red line) and of the ECMWF data in analysis (continuous blue line). (Color figure online)

anticipated, a direct comparison between the measured and the hindcast data is not correct. Hence, in order to perform a proper comparison between the measured wind data and computed ones, the analysis, previously described, has been used to estimate the actual heeling angle $\overline{\alpha}$, and consequently to quantify the changes in the measurement height z. Note that a similar approach has been shown in [8], nevertheless since at that time no information on the real heeling of the boat were available, then just a parametric analysis of the heeling angle was performed.

As qualitatively shown in Fig. 9, the heeling angle α modifies the measurement height to be used in the Eq. (3). The lower panel of the Fig. 13 shows the results of the comparison between the measured wind data and the numerical ones (i.e. GFS and ECMWF). In this case, Eq. (3) has been used by assuming for the heeling angle $\overline{\alpha}$ (see upper panel of Fig. 13, red line). It appears that the comparison between the measured wind data (black line) and the numerical ones (both those obtained by using the GFS and the ECMWF) improves. Nevertheless, it is worth noticing that the measured wind data exhibit the maximum discrepancy from the numerical ones as the peak of the storms occurs.

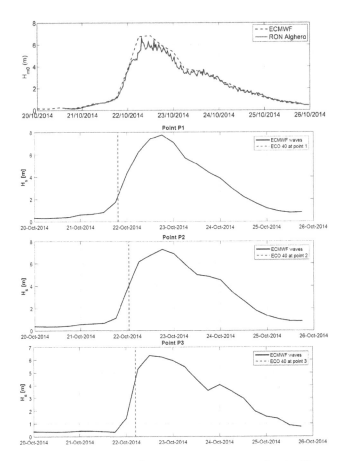

Fig. 14. First panel (i.e. upper panel): comparison between the significant wave height H_s measured by the Alghero buoy and the same quantity obtained from the analysis data of the ECMWF. Remaining panels (i.e. second, third and fourth): evolution over time of the significant wave height Hs, as obtained from the numerical model of the ECMWF, evaluated in three points of interest placed along the route of the boat. Note: the vertical dashed red lines identify the time at which the boat has passed in that point. (Color figure online)

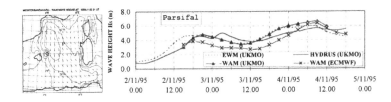

Fig. 15. Significant wave height time series during the Gulf of Lions storm of 2 November 1995 that has caused the sinking of the Parsifal (Figs. 5 and 6 of the paper of [3]).

This discrepancy can be explained by looking at the middle panel of the Fig. 13. It shows the analysis data (ECMWF) of the significant wave height H_s interpolated (in time and space) along the route of the boat between Sardinia Island and the Balearic Islands. As the peak of the storm occurs, then the significant wave height H_s faced by ECO40 is in the order of 5 m (see Sect. 6). It implies that, by assuming the waves Rayleigh distributed, then a maximum wave height $H_{max} \simeq 1.8 * H_s$ equal to about 9 m may be experienced by the boat. Therefore, we can assume that the coefficient C_{10} in the Eq. (3), that is function of the flow regime of the wind speed and of the surface roughness that depends on the waves conditions, is not well estimated in such rough wave conditions. Furthermore, Fig. 13 shows that, as the time increases (over 60 h), the agreement between the forecast data and the measured ones deteriorates.

6   Wave Data Analysis

This section briefly describes the analysis carried out on the wave data collected during the Gulf of Lions event. The available wave data sources are: the buoy of Alghero (Italy), that is part of the RON (Italian National Network for the wave measurements; see [10]) and the data provided by the numerical model of the ECMWF. Figure 14 shows the time series of the significant wave height Hs in few points of interest placed along the route of the boat. The upper panel shows the comparison between the significant wave height Hs measured by the Alghero buoy and the Hs obtained by linearly interpolating the data provided in analysis by ECMWF (dashed line). The two set of data are in good agreement: indeed both the shape and the maximum values appear quite similar. The remaining panels (second, third and fourth) show the evolution over time of the significant wave height Hs, as obtained from the numerical model of the ECMWF, evaluated in three points of interest (P1: 40.50, 6.50; P2: 40.25, 5.75; P3: 39.75, 5.00) placed along the route of the boat. The vertical dashed red lines identify the time at which the boat has passed in that point and therefore show the values of the significant wave height experienced by the boat. Note that, in the future, such numerical wave data will be compared with the ones obtained by the signals measured by the three high-precision GPS.

Finally, Fig. 15 shows the significant wave height time series during the Gulf of Lions storm of November 1995 that has been reconstructed by [3]. We recall that this storm caused the sinking of the Italian sailboat Parsifal and the death of 6 crew members. Although a quantitative comparison is not actually possible here, we can qualitatively assess that the magnitude of the sea state that ECO40 has faced is quite comparable with that suffered by the Parsifal.

7   Concluding Remarks and Ongoing Research

This paper analyses, both in terms of the met-ocean conditions and in terms of the boat heeling, the first violent storm experienced by ECO40 during its navigation that occurred in the Gulf of Lion on October 21–22, 2014. The heeling of the boat has been estimated by using the GPS signals that have been analyzed by using a moving base kinematic approach. This analysis has allowed to estimate the heeling angle α during the whole storm event. As far as the met-ocean conditions are concerned, the storm has been analysed on the basis of the wind data, averaged over 10 min, measured and transmitted almost in real time from the boat. These wind data have compared with the ones obtained by using two numerical models: the forecast data as from the GFS and the analysis data as from the ECMWF. This comparison, along with the results of the heeling analysis, has shown that the wind measurement height (z) plays an important role. The corrected measurements of the wind, averaged over 10 min, are comparable with the results obtained from the numerical models: a good agreement is noticeable within the first 60 h. Nevertheless, a sensible discrepancy between the measured wind data and the numerical one is noticeable as the storm peak occurs. This discrepancy may be referred to the "large roughness" of the sea surface (i.e. severe wave conditions) that in our opinion is not well caught by the used theoretical model of the wind velocity vertical profile. As the time increases, then the numerical results tend to deteriorate. Furthermore, the forecast data seem to well predict not only the magnitude of the event, in terms of wind speed, but also the exact time of occurrence of the storm peak, a parameter often prone to error. The direct comparison between the forecast and the measured wind speed showed, in the present case (anemometer located at the nominal height of +19.0 m above m.s.l.), as expected, relevant discrepancies. These discrepancies are such to underestimate the forecast wind condition in the order of 50% of the forecast wind for severe storm conditions. These differences are due to: (i) the differences in the height at which wind measurements are carried out which are estimated to yield in the present case almost a 35% error for strong wind and (ii) the gust (approximately a 15% error). In this context it is important to highlight that the sail trim on board is carried out by using "reference wind condition" which normally are related to the true wind speed and direction measured on board by means of the anemometer located on the top of the mast. The obtained results show that for sailboats having the mast length greater than +10 m, it is very important to adequately increase the wind speed forecast in order to obtain a safe prediction.

Finally, we presented qualitative comparison between the present wave data (obtained from the RON buoy of Alghero and from the ECMWF analysis data) and those reconstructed by [3] that refer to the storm of November 1995 that caused the sinking of Parsifal. We have found a substantial similarity in terms of sea-state magnitude between the two events.

Furthermore, it is worth noticing that in the future a comparison between the measured wave data, as obtained by the signals measured by the three high-precision GPS placed on the sailboat, and the ones obtained from the available source of wave data (e.g. numerical models, remote sensing techniques, wave buoys, etc.) will be performed.

Acknowledgements. The authors would like to acknowledge Dr. Pier Paolo Pecoraro (IDROGEOTEC) for his expertise and help during the installation of the instruments. The skipper Matteo Miceli is also acknowledged for his contribution. A special acknowledgement is due to Leica Geosystem for providing the high-precision GPS reveivers. A warm acknowledgment is due to Eng. Francesco Farina which has developed the navigation software Smart Skipper, including the feature for sending the metocean data to the land team.

References

1. Benedetti, E., Branzanti, M., Biagi, L., Colosimo, G., Mazzoni, A., Crespi, M.: Global navigation satellite systems seismology for the 2012 mw 6.1 emilia earthquake: exploiting the vadase algorithm. Seismol. Res. Lett. **85**(3), 649–656 (2014)
2. Benedetti, E., Branzanti, M., Colosimo, G., Mazzoni, A., Crespi, M.: Vadase: state of the art and new developments of a third way to gnss seismology (2015)
3. Bertotti, L., Cavaleri, L., De Girolamo, P., Franco, L., Magnaldi, S.: Hindcast and forecast of the parsifal storm. Nuovo cimento della Società italiana di fisica. C **21**(3), 281–298 (1998)
4. Branzanti, M., Colosimo, G., Crespi, M., Mazzoni, A.: Gps near-real-time coseismic displacements for the great tohoku-oki earthquake. IEEE Geosci. Remote Sens. Lett. **10**(2), 372–376 (2013)
5. Colosimo, G., Crespi, M., Mazzoni, A.: Real-time GPS seismology with a standalone receiver: A preliminary feasibility demonstration. J. Geophys. Res. **116**, B11302 (2011). doi:10.1029/2010JB007941
6. Colosimo, G., Crespi, M., Mazzoni, A., Dautermann, T.: Co-seismic displacement estimation: Improving tsunami early warning systems. GIM Int. **25**, 19–23 (2011)
7. Crespi, M., Mazzoni, A., Colosimo, G.: Global and local reference frames. Rendiconti Lincei, pp. 1–7 (2015)
8. De Girolamo, P., Romano, A., Pezzoli, A., Boscolo, A., Crespi, M., Mazzoni, A., Di Risio, M., Pasquali, D., Franco, L., Sammarco, P.: Analysis of the 21/22 october 2014 storm experienced by the sailboat eco40 in the gulf of lion. In: Proceedings of the International Congress on Sport Sciences Research and Technology Support, icSPORTS 2015, pp. 290–298 (2015)
9. Pierson, W.J.: Wind generated gravity waves. Adv. Geophys. **2**, 93–178 (1955)
10. Piscopia, R., Inghilesi, R., Panizzo, A., Corsini, S., Franco, L.: Analysis of 12-year wave measurements by the Italian wave network. In: Coastal Engineering Conference, vol. 1, pp. 121–133. World Scientific (2002)
11. Takasu, T.: Rtklib: Open source program package for rtk-gps. In: Proceedings of the FOSS4G (2009)
12. Wu, J.: Froude number scaling of wind-stress coefficients. J. Atmos. Sci. **26**(3), 408–413 (1969)

Tactical Skills Training in Team Sports: Technological Supports for the 4P Strategy

Gilles Kermarrec[1,2(✉)]

[1] Research Center for Education, Learning and Didactics,
UEB University, Brest, France
gilles.kermarrec@univ-brest.fr
[2] European Center for Virtual Reality, Plouzané, France

Abstract. Since few years decision-making in team sports has been studied through a Naturalistic Decision-Making (NDM) approach. Considering the need for an intuitive and coordinated decision-making (ICDM), implications from NDM framework are examined according to literature on tactical skills training in team sports. Small-Sided Games (SSGs) are approved by a large majority of coach and researchers. Nevertheless, the pedagogical use of SSG led to implicit learning according to the Led-Constraints framework, whereas it focused on explicit learning according to the Teaching-Games-For-Understanding model. According to NDM, there is a need for a wide range of decision-making processes in team sports, so that a tactical skills training strategy should be based on a blend of implicit and explicit learning. Thus, scientists and coaches in soccer designed the 4P strategy (i.e., Positioning; Practicing; Picturing; Post-analysing). Complementary they explored the role of technology supports embedded into the 4P strategy. Results suggested that soccer players benefited from video feedback because it highlighted relevant configurations of play and helped them to share "pictures" during small-sided games.

Keywords: Naturalistic Decision-Making · Intuition · Coordination · Training · Small-sided games · Implicit vs explicit learning · Technology supports · Video feedback

1 Introduction

Over the past three decades research in sport sciences has focused on the "winning factors" such as tactical skills. Whereas strategic competence reflects the capability to plan an action, tactical skill is the capability to make relevant choices within the course of an action [1]. Thus, tactical skills can be viewed as a blend of automatic and deliberated processes, a blend of motoric – emotional – perceptive and cognitive factors, a blend of individual and collective response to a complex and dynamic situation. The purpose of this chapter is to examine the implications of sport sciences research for tactical skills training. How should coaches design training sessions? Which kind of feedbacks should help players to improve their tactical skills? Could new technologies be a support for such training?

© Springer International Publishing AG 2016
J. Cabri and P. Pezarat Correia (Eds.): icSPORTS 2015, CCIS 632, pp. 106–125, 2016.
DOI: 10.1007/978-3-319-52770-3_8

Findings in sports sciences offer a large set of arguments for the interest of small-sided games (SSG) especially for tactical skills training in soccer [2]. SSG is not only a reduced game, but also we consider it as a combination of coaches' objective and task constraints: "space (e.g., the nature of the playing surface, playing area dimensions), time (e.g., time span of matches, time to attain a sub-objective of the match), players (e.g., number of players in each team, number of teams, roles of players), equipment (e.g., size and number of goals and balls), and intrapersonal and interpersonal coordination (e.g., limbs allowed to contact the ball or players allowed to pass the ball)". Practicing SSG is supposed to involve a large set of capabilities, such as physiological, technical or tactical capabilities in soccer.

The use of small-sided games for tactical skills training is viewed as an archetype of the constraints-led approach of training [2]. The manipulation of human and environmental constraints is supposed to shape players behaviours. Researchers demonstrated that games, called Small-Sided-Conditioned-Games (SSCG), could enhance individual and collective tactical skills [3]. This research program and its implications are arisen from the Ecological Dynamics (ED) approach. In this perspective tactical skills emerge from the interactions of individuals with environmental constraints and SSCGs provoke behaviour adaptations and implicit learning.

Small-sided games are approved by a large majority of coaches and scientists for tactical skills training in soccer. For practitioners, SSGs promote "true experiences"; for scientists, SSG are relevant because they are "authentic" [4], or because they are "representative" [3]. Nevertheless, very recent papers pointed that key distinctions between theoretical backgrounds for SSGs exist and that it should have implications for « the pedagogical use of SSG » [5, 6]. It is not clear how and why coaches and teachers should in help players in modifying their behaviour within SSGs. Thus, there is a need for a better understanding about the effects of task's constraints on decision-making learning and about the effects of coaches' interventions within the games. Does behaviours' changes relied on changes in decision-making processes? Which constraint provokes effect on decision-making learning? How coaches could help players when tactical skills need spontaneous and accurate decision-making? In recent times, decision-making in a sport setting began to be studied through a Naturalistic Decision-Making (NDM) approach. We made the assumption that advances from this framework could provide principles in order to improve the "pedagogical use of SSG" in tactical skills training sessions.

The Naturalistic Decision-Making paradigm (Klein, 1998–2008) investigates how people make choices and coordinate themselves in military, nuclear power, aviation, human management, economic or sports settings [7]. More specifically, NDM examines the ways in which experts in real-world contexts, alone or in a team, identify and assess situations, make decisions and coordinate their actions. NDM is a theoretical and methodological perspective from ergonomic psychology, and its expected outcomes are both of better understanding of decision-making in teams and improving training devices or teaching methods. For that, we made the assumption that NDM advances could be helpful for tactical skills training in team sports.

This chapter aims at presenting an innovative tactical skills training strategy called the 4P Strategy. The 4P strategy was based on recent advances from NDM in team sports. First, we overview findings from our research on team performances. The results provide a rationale for targeting Intuitive and Coordinated Decision-Making (ICDM) in team sports, and have implications for designing decision-making training. Second, these insights lead scientists and practitioners to design the 4P strategy, the principles of which are presented and illustrated. Third, the 4P tactical skills training strategy has been experimented within technological supports; we brought proofs that technological supports embedded in naturalistic training devices provide precious help for players.

2   Tactical Skills in Team Sports: Advances from the NDM Perspective

2.1   Tactical Skills and Intuitive Decision-Making: The RPD Model

The NDM approach emphases an intuitive decision-making. The intuitive decision-making is an alternative to the rationalistic linear information-processing model. Rationalistic or analytic decision-making refers to a relatively slow and conscious process, so that it could not be effective in many sport situations.

Klein (1998–2008) has shown that experts in dynamic situations do not tend to make decisions based on rational deductions or exhaustive analyses of expectancies. Contrariwise, intuitive decision-making supposed that people confronted with uncertainty and time pressure are able to perceive relevant cues in the context and to recognize the configuration of a situation as typical. This recognition process is sufficient to adjust behaviour to the particular conditions of the environment through typical actions. The Recognition-Primed Decision [7] model suggests three levels of experiencing the situation: simple matching if the situation is quickly perceived as familiar; diagnosis when the situation is perceived to be incongruous; simulation when an expert perceives the situation as typical and has time for assessing his option through mental simulation before implementing a course of action.

RPD models started to be applied also in sport settings over the last years (for a brief review, see [8]). Most of the studies used a video-cued interview and a "first person approach" in a competitive setting. The results in Table 1 confirmed that experts in sport games recognize configuration of a play and made decisions based on previous experiences:

(a) They only perceived the most salient informational cues of a situation, and matched them together to recognized typical configurations of play. These cues are visual cues in context, expected goals, and available motoric skills, more than explicit knowledge. Most of the time, the configuration of play recognition relies on distances, positions, and movement, speed: it's a spatiotemporal configuration.

(b) They tend to use a simple match mechanism and take the first option when they assessed the situations as familiar; simple matching was the most relevant mechanism in offensive phases, and especially in counter-attacks.

(c) When players did not assess the situation as familiar, two or more rarely three options were diagnosed. During defending phases the players did not initiate the game and because and they felt the uncertainty of the situation, they compared two options.

Table 1. RPD model in sports settings: frequencies of recognition process players used in different team sports (percentages are put into brackets). Adapted from Kermarrec & Bossard [8].

RPD model in sport settings	Volley-ball Macquet (2009)	Ice-hockey Bossard et al. (2010)	Ice-hockey Mulligan et al. (2012)	Soccer Kermarrec & Bossard (2014)	Handball Le Menn & Kermarrec (2015)
Sequences or stages	Attack and defence in the same stage	Counter-attacks	Experts in attack stages	Defensive stage	Goalkeeper: Shooting sequences
Simple match	57/70 (0.81)	46/57 (0.80)	68/80 (0.85)	68/112 0.60	38/83 (0.46)
Simulate	4/70 (0.07)	2/57 (0.03)		26/112 (0.23)	28/83 (0.34)
Diagnose	9/70 (0.12)	9/57 (0.17)	16/80 (0.15)	18/112 (0.16)	17/83 (0.20)

(d) When players did not feel urgency, they took time to simulate the situation: especially defenders or goalkeeper anticipated opponents' options when they were far from the ball. They evaluate the situation from their own internal "first person" viewpoint, or from an external "third person" viewpoint. Especially the goal-keeper tried to imagine the shooting player's options, from his own point of view. This process allows him or her to evaluate how effective the defensive options will be in the current situation.

(e) The more the players are experimented, the more they tend to make a typical choice; recognition and action relied on typical schemas, which are the outcomes of training and previous experiences.

Finally, empirical studies pointed out evidences for intuitive decision-making used by experts in team sports. In other words, according to NDM approach, tactical skills rely on recognition of typical configurations of play. In next section we examine tactical skills as a collective capability, and the need to share the same configuration of play in order to make coordinated decision-making.

2.2 Tactical Skills and Coordinated Decision-Making: The TSA Model

In NDM perspective, team performance requires a high degree of coordination. Thus, NDM line of research on team performances has shown the interest of the Team Situation Awareness (TSA). TSA is a well-known model used to better understand coordination in teams [9, 10].

In dynamic and complex situations like most team games interactions, coordination between teammates cannot be reduced to a strategy and a plan. Knowledge constructed and shared before the course of action (i.e., Shared Mental Models) are not sufficient. Because tactical skills cannot be reduced to strategic competences, team members have to share perceptions, judgements, expectations during the on-going situation. Considering that what is shared could be "contextual", some researchers have developed conceptual and methodological frameworks for describing and assessing the dynamic of coordination. In this regard, the notion of situation awareness was extended to study coordination in teams. Endsley (1995) defined Situation Awareness as the perception of the elements in the context, the understanding of their meaning, and the projection of their role in the near future [11]. In other words, SA is a "picture" of a situation to which it refers [12]. Over the past few years, Team Situation Awareness (TSA) has emerged as a major concept in research dedicated to study coordination among members of the same team. Both of quantitative and qualitative methods were employed. TSA was assessed with a particular focus on the shared contents, on the forms of sharing that appeared during real-time activity, and on the sharing processes.

We conducted a study in Handball [13] from the TSA perspective. Behavioural data from six elite players during offensive phases were recorded and supplemented by verbal data collected during video-cued recall interviews after the game. Content analysis was conducted. The results showed that the athletes alternated between two modes of coordination. In some cases, a pre-established plan was followed-up, based on shared content or "sharedness" (e.g. the routines or tactics that were reinforced during training). Most of the time, these shared content have to be adjusted at the end of the course of action. In other cases, performances needed a real-time adaptation to the context of action. "Context sharing" during the course of action is based on a dynamic process of sharing a configuration of a play. Complementary, many sharing processes such as inquiry or surveying, verifying or monitoring, displaying, masking or resisting authorized members of team to adjust their own decision to ones' decision, or to influence ones' decision.

This study elicited the alternative role of knowledge sharedness (as a "static plan") and configuration of a play sharing (as a "dynamic process in context"). Considering that sharedness is rarely sufficient and completely pre-established before team performance, most of the recent studies from the TSA perspective pointed out that training methods have to develop further in the direction of team adaptation [10]. Thus team-training strategies should target "team work" rather than "task work" [14]. Whereas task work consisted essentially in explicit learning occurring in pre-briefing or post-briefing, team work emphases the role of practice and implicit learning, and the need for sharing within the course of action. In this perspective tactical skills training in team sports could consist in involving the capabilities for players to recognize and share the same configurations of play during the on-going situation.

To conclude this brief report on advances from the NDM perspective, empirical findings lead us to modelling tactical skill in team sports as an intuitive and coordinated decision-making (ICDM). RPD model and TSA models are gathered together in the above in order to describe players' macrocognitive activity (sharing, learning), the by-products the players use (environmental cues, typical actions, plausible goals, etc.), the recognition processes (simple match, diagnosing, simulation), and the outcomes from experiences (typical schemas). Thus, we suggest that tactical skills models should consider both of individual and collective capabilities, and that tactical skills training should focus on *configuration of play recognition and sharing* Fig. 1.

3 Enhancing Intuitive and Coordinated Decision-Making: The 4P Strategy

Despite many studies emphasise the interest of the NDM approach to better understand the mechanism underlying expertise in team sports, very few have inspired decision-making training tools in a sports setting [5].

According to NDM perspective, tactical skills need and configuration of play recognition need a large range of individual mechanisms depending on both the familiarity of the situation and time pressure: simple match when the situation is usual; diagnosing when the situation is unclear; simulating and evaluating when time pressure is not too high. Klein [7] claimed that intuitive decision-making should be trained through four key ways: (a) engaging in realistic practice; (b) compiling extensive experiences; (c) obtaining accurate and quick feedbacks; (d) reviewing prior experiences and learning from mistakes. Complementary, Hogarth [15] has developed a learning approach to intuition. First, environments in which intuitions are trained need to be representative for the environments in which intuitions are supposed to be applied. Second, he highlighted the role of feedback that should be speedy, accurate and relevant. He pointed out that learners do not need explicit feedback, explanations, or conscious awareness of the on-going learning situation. Hogarth's assumptions have been widely accepted in the field of intuition research.

An earlier application of an intuitive decision-making approach has been developed based on the Ecological Rationality perspective [1]. This perspective describes "the match between a decision-making strategy and the environment in which it is used"

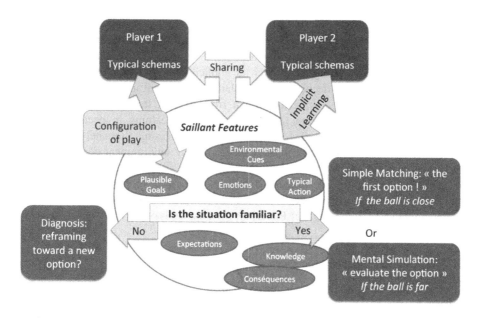

Fig. 1. The ICDM model in team sports: a tactical skills model from NDM perspective.

Training Models	TGfU	4P Strategy	SMART	LCA
Coaches Interventions	Verbal Feedbacks	Video Feedbacks	Automatic feedbacks from environment	
Learning Continuum	Explicit	← ———————————————— →		**Implicit**
Learning processes	*Analysing, Debating, Verbalizing, Co-constructing*	*Configuration of Play Recognition Picturing Sharing in Context*	*Behaviours emergence Affordances Perception Co-adaptation*	
Decision-Making Models	**Knowledge-Based Shared Mental Models**	**Ecological Rationality RPD & TSA (NDM)**	**Ecological Dynamics**	

Fig. 2. Tactical Skills Training Models and their frameworks.

(id., p. 4). Because the relevant choices depend on constraints in environment, a large range of decision-making mechanisms is available, and none model of decision-making should be considered as superior to other.

Thus, Raab [1] suggested that explicit or implicit learning should be promoted taking in account the complexity of the training task. In line with the Ecological Rationality framework, a tactical skills training model, called SMART (Situation Model of Anticipated Response consequences of Tactical Training) promotes the use of implicit leaning in low-complexity task, and explicit learning in high complexity task. In games, explicit learning is promoted when the learner is guided in analysing, debating, self – evaluating (e.g. the Teaching Games for Understanding Model [4]). In contrary, the Led-Constraints Approach [2] promotes implicit learning, because the actions of individual players or interpersonal interactions between players are supposed to emerge from the coupling between players and the task constraints. Implicit learning relies on behaviour adaptation without being aware to the knowledge underlying task achievement, whereas explicit learning relies on analysis and verbalization in order to construct rules or knowledge about the task. Thus, tactical skills training models (see Fig. 2) could be placed along the explicit *vs* implicit learning continuum [1, 5].

Theoretically intuitive decision-making claims for implicit learning. Nevertheless, practically it is difficult to separate implicit from explicit learning within learners' experiences in training program. The role of explicit learning in decision-making training is not clear. Whereas SMART model suggested using alternately implicit or explicit learning, we argued that in naturalistic training environment coaches should use a wide range of artefacts for decision-making training, including both of implicit and explicit learning. In line with this rationale, a team of sport scientists and professional coaches in soccer designed the 4P strategy. It's a four-step-strategy: (a) Positioning; (b) Practicing; (c) Picturing; (d) Post-analysing.

3.1   Positioning the Training Device

Positioning the training device within a realistic performance context consists in introducing a tactical objective in line with previous performances. In other words coaches should use prebriefing as a way toward the sense of the game.

This principle is consistent with the heart of the TGFU approach [4]: a technical or tactical objective should be only introduced if the players can make sense about it, or can feel the need for it when they have performed a real game. From the NDM approach, this principle is led on the sensemaking assumption. In team sport sensemaking is a continuous process of understanding the play. Sensemaking is a retrospective analysis of events and a projection to the future. The Frame Theory of sensemaking brought interesting implications for learning and training. A frame, call it schema, map, story or script, helps us to recognize, connect or filter data in the environment [8].

Positioning the training device consists in facilitating the framing process of coupling within the game environment. Framing should be supported when an objective is positioned in the on-going "history" of a team (previous and future competition matches), positioned in specific sub-phases of team games (such as preparing the attempt to the goal, defending a zone, or passing the ball from the defenders to the forwards), and concretely positioned in a space on the field.

3.2 Practicing SSPG

Practicing Small-Sided-Positioned Games is a consequence of previous step. The focus is made on designing realistic or representative small-sided games that could implicitly shape configurations of play required for competitive team games performance. This principle seems to be consistent with theoretical advances (i.e., representative design) and empirical findings from the CLA [3]. Therefore, it is based on some arguments from the NDM line of research.

First, empirical studies showed that recognition mechanisms experts used depend on their position on the standard competitive pitch [8]. We suggest that the location of the small-sided game within the standard pitch could enhance the representativeness of a game. In other words, sense making in the game and configuration recognition may depend on the on-field location within the standard pitch. Thus position of the game must be thought in accordance with the configuration of play the coach wants to be trained.

Second, because intuitive decision-making is based on a spatiotemporal recognition, our results pointed out that timing is relevant when experts identified a configuration of a play (id.); SSG could simulate specific sub-phases of team games such as preparing the attempt to the goal, defending a zone, or passing the ball from the defenders to the forwards. Especially each time a play is ended (e.g. the ball get out of the playing area), a game's starter should throw again the ball in the same area in order to lead to cumulative experiences.

Third, because previous research on decision-making in team sports demonstrated that spatiotemporal recognition is based on the players' point of view, the players' positions in the game should be related to their own position or task in their competitive team. In SSG each time the game starts again, the players should go back to their assigned positions in the game.

All of these points lead us to the idea that SSGs should be Small-Sided Positioned Games (SSPGs); a SSPG and a classical SSG are illustrated in Figs. 3 and 4.

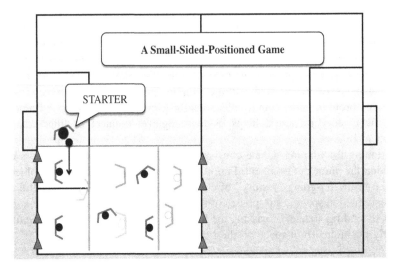

Fig. 3. An example of a SSPG aiming at passing the ball from the defenders to the forwards.

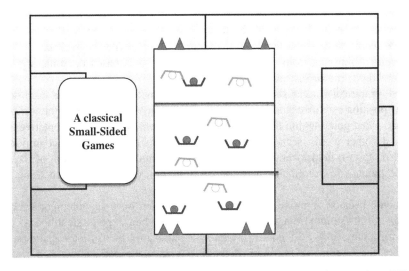

Fig. 4. An example of a classical SSG presenting the same structure than previous SSPG.

3.3 Picturing the Expected Configuration of Play

In order to highlight configuration of play, the coach can use the "Stop, Watch and Go" pedagogical artefact in SSPG [16]: he stops the game shortly, orders the players to stay in place, stresses them to briefly watch their relations or positions, notes if the configuration is expected or not, and starts the play again. Because "picturing the configuration of play" is based on visual chunks more than on verbal information, this step of the 4P strategy should be classify more toward the pole of implicit learning than explicit learning. Of course in the field both types of learning are present [1].

This step is driven from NDM empirical findings. Studies based on RPD model highlighted the role of spatiotemporal configuration recognition in intuitive decision-making. These configurations are a blend of distances, visual cues, goals, and available motoric skills, more than explicit knowledge. The aim of this pedagogical step is also to help players, players and coach, to share, and to reinforce or to throw out the same picture, when the team failed or succeed [12].

3.4   Post-analysing the Game

Post-analysing the game is not only a debriefing, aiming at evaluating and providing explicit feedbacks. It is also a time for putting pictures into words and concepts, for debating choices that players have made, for associating configuration of play and knowledge or tactical principles, and for sharing them between players and coaches. This principle seems to be consistent with theoretical advances and empirical findings from the TGFU approach: language productions, debate ideas about action and strategies are supposed to produce an impact on explicit learning [4].

This fourth step of our 4P strategy is also based on some arguments from the NDM line of research. Promoting verbal exchanges between players should improve their cognitive package for future decision-making. In work field, debriefing is a key point for improving individual decision-making [7] and for team coordination [9]. In a sport setting, recent findings suggested that expert defenders [8] used knowledge to diagnose or simulate the situation, when the ball is far from them. Post-analysing the game is a key point for coaches in order to organize schemata within scripts or global frames, in order to classify specific configuration of play into a whole defensive or offensive strategy, in accordance with a game style or philosophy.

Findings from NDM researches in team sport, led to designing a 4P strategy. In next section, we present how coaches have experimented the 4P strategy. Furthermore, technologies supports have integrated within the 4P strategy, and effects on tactical skills were expected.

4   Technology Supports Within the 4P Strategy

In the world of high performance sport, and especially in team sports, elite coaches are increasingly tapping into the world of technology and innovation. In many ways, the emerging area of the 'technology driven sport space' is changing both the way that we practice and the way we train. The question is: will new technologies take the place of traditional training device, or will technological supports reinforce actual training device efficacy? The potential benefits of new technologies have led many researchers to develop research programmes relating to computer simulation, virtual reality, video-based learning, video feedback, etc. … But, although simulations in the fields of driving, aviation and military or medical interventions is no longer questioned, there is very little information available about the benefits of simulations for research and training in sports [17].

For instance, virtual reality simulation, that is to say performing an action outside of its regular context, is supposed to serve many purposes in the context of high-level sports: preparing oneself for action, acquiring new technical skills, or studying particular techniques. The transfer of skills from the simulation to reality is considered as a measure of the simulation's success as a training tool. Some experimental studies have shown effective skills transfer, while others have shown less significant results (for a complete review of these tests, see [18]). Thus there is need for research and development that will connect practitioners, engineers and researchers in order to significantly improve training effectiveness while reducing its costs.

This challenge is driven by a combination of new technologies and emerging trends in learning, including video-based training as a second example of new technologies potential. A body of research in sports sciences has used video as a means of measuring and training perceptual and decision-making skills in a variety of sports. Expert-novice studies using a video occlusion method have shown that expert athletes are able to make better and earlier recognition of an opponent's action. Nevertheless very few studies have measured transfer of video training to real game performance (see [19]).

Reviews on the interest of new technologies for training, in cognitive psychology [18], and in sport science [17], have shown that acquisitions are linked to the context and that transfer of learning was hypothetical. This provides a rationale for considering that technology supports should be seemed as artefacts integrated in real world training devices. In this section, we advocated that technology supports embedded within the 4P strategy are potentially effective resources for coaches.

4.1   The Potential of Technological Supports for Training Tactical Skills

Technology can provide effective support for tactical skills training, because it can be helpful for both of the coaching process and the learning process. To our mind, new technology can be supports performance analysis and performance feedbacks.

Performance analysis in sport sciences relies on notational analysis and on motion analysis (see Fig. 5). Notational analysis provides factual record about the position of the ball, the players involved, the action concerned, the time and the outcome of the activity. Such data and consequent analysis can be applied to select objectives for training session. More specifically, they can help the coach for *positioning* the training device in relationship with team's performance in previous competition. Motion analysis focuses on movement of the ball, a player, or the whole team. For instance, player tracking systems such as Prozone can collect distance covered, number of sprints and high-intensity distance covered, indicating aspects of the activity during of match play which can be use within the coaching process to devise training sessions related to specific tactical problem. The detail provided by these systems allows the identification of specific needs, and furnishes factual features for coaches in order to engage their players toward an objective or a training task such as a SSPG.

Complementary, notational analysis and motion analysis can lead to performance modelling. Performance modelling consists in reducing performance complexity into

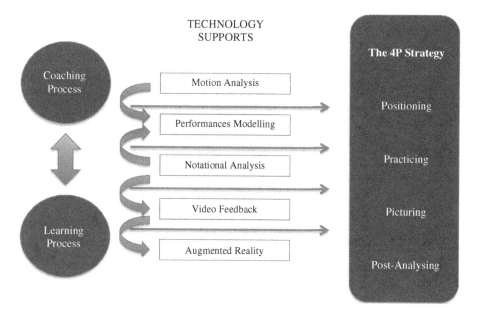

Fig. 5. The potential of technological supports for coaching and learning.

symbolic, graphic, mathematic representation. In so doing, modelling is supposed to focus attention on a specific aspect of performance, or to favour shared understanding of performance factors. Performance modelling works as a mirror of individuals or teams' own activity, participates in *picturing*, and can involve the learning process.

Video feedback works also as a mirror from previous experiences. The use of video feedback is one of the most frequently cited technologies that researchers suggest may have the most impact within learning process in sport and physical education [20]. Concretely, video technology support can be facilitated through use of slow motion, live capture, and instant replay aiming at furnishing an accurate and immediate feedback. For instance, in soccer, Groom, Cushion & Nelson [21] highlighted the potential of video analysis as a training tool due to the detailed and clear nature of performance feedback. In this perspective, video feedbacks may help players to evaluate behavioural aspects of performance such as individuals' errors or coordination between teammates. Furthermore, video technology can be used within the "picturing step" of the 4P strategy. Nevertheless it is well known that the more immediate is a feedback the more efficient it is for learning and there remain a number of practical challenges for researchers and coaches. Thus we suggest that the advent of technologies such as tablet devices made it more manageable for *picturing* configurations of play.

Digital video technology derives to augmented reality when displaying relevant information. For instance, some camera (e.g., Go Pro hero 4) have the ability to allow you to mark specific moments in your video; for instance a soccer coach can highlight relationships between the players, the ball, and the position of the game (i.e., a configuration of play). This kind of video augmented feedback can be provided when the coach stops the game and helps players to "picture" the relevant configuration of play.

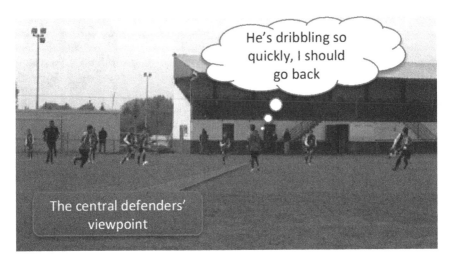

Fig. 6. An example of displaying a teammate viewpoint within a defensive team.

Video tagging can also be convenient for post-analysing a game. For instance, Kermarrec & Bossard [22] have experimented such a video feedback in order to enhance shared understanding in youth players' team. Their findings supported the idea that an innovative 2-D video feedback, using viewpoint changes and displaying teammates' judgments, should enhance shared understanding between four defensive players during *post-analysing* session (Fig. 6)

Finally, the potential of technology for coaching and learning relies on a need for more and more information about the winning factors underlying the game. Technology supports provide both of quantitative and qualitative data, quantitative through the application of statistical analysis of team and player performance, qualitative through the use of video. Video feedbacks relate to technical, tactical, individual or collective, aspects of team sports. In order to systematically experiment and assess the potential of technology support within the 4P strategy, a cooperative research program have been conducted, gathering together professional coaches and researchers from the Brittany Soccer League in France. It was expected that the 4P strategy and video feedbacks were well suited for intuitive and coordinated decision-making training. Two recent studies are presented in next sections.

4.2   Effect of Video Feedback on Intuitive Decision-Making

A first study was designed in order to investigate the 4P strategy's effect on individual recognition of configuration of play in youth players [23]. Video-cued artefacts were introduced; it was expected that it could support recognition processes within the third step of the 4P strategy. *Picturing* consisted in stopping the game for a very short time when a relevant configuration emerges from the on-going situation, watching the configuration and focusing attention on relevant cues, and going on the game. It was hypothesized that technological device such as digital tablet could support picturing

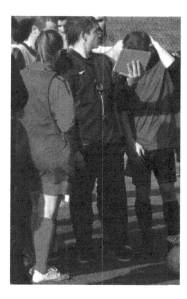

Fig. 7. Picturing a configuration of play through digital tablet device.

and recognition of relevant configurations of play. The video of the game was recorded through digital camera, and immediately sent to the tablet thanks to Bluetooth system (see Fig. 7).

Setting and Participants. The 4P strategy and video feedbacks were experimented in four soccer schools (U13) from the Brittany soccer League in France. Forty youth players (mean ± SD; age = 12,53 ± 1.62) participated in this study, divided by 4 groups depending to their own soccer school. For each group the objective of training sequence was to be able to better transport the ball from the defenders to the attackers. Each group had 10 players who were divided into two teams of 5 players each by the coaches. Players and their parents were fully informed of aims and procedures of the study and signed a consent form.

Procedure. First, each group played a classical SSG (see Fig. 4) at the beginning of the usual training session on a 30 × 50 m pitch with 10 min duration (pre-test). Then, the four groups practiced two periods of 15 min (training conditions), and a recovery period of 5 min between them. Each group had a specific condition. Three groups practiced a specific SSPG (see Fig. 3) aiming at enhancing the advance of the ball from the defenders to the attackers within a team. The area for both SSG and SSPG was a 50 × 30 m rectangle divided into 3 areas. The players are divided into two teams, which play 5 *vs* 5. Each team is allowed to score in any of their 2 goals. In the SSPG, the players are positioned within the inner zones depending on their tasks in the team (2 defenders, 2 midfielders, 1 forward). The game starts with the team positioned in the defense zone, when the starter passes the ball to one of the defender. The goal is to advance the ball in the field and score in one of the two targets. If the opponents get the ball, they also try to score a goal in any of their 2 goals.

Conditions. The four training conditions were: C1, practicing the classical SSG; C2, practicing the SSPG, without any specific verbal instruction or demonstration; C3, practicing the SSPG and furnishing pedagogical aids through the 4P strategy; C4, practicing the SSPG and furnishing pedagogical aids though the 4P strategy included video feedbacks.

Data Collection. All the games were videotaped from a fixed and high position. Video-recorded images were transferred to a digital support for analyses. We tracked the ball position on the screen and measured the *Ball Advance* (i.e., the advance of the ball from the defenders to the attackers within each team's possession of the ball, in meters). Researchers and coaches considered the *Ball Advance* as a good indicator for learning assessment. Each time the player recognized an opportunity to pass the ball toward the next zone, and made the relevant choice, the ball was carried some meters longer toward the goal. It was considered as an objective measure of tactical skills learning, in line with pedagogical content (i.e., being able to transport the ball from the defenders to the attackers).

Data Analysis. Distances' measure method was inspired by the method using a single camera and combining manual video tracking and bi-dimensional reconstruction for sports performance analysis (Duarte et al., 2010). Virtual distances data (i.e., pixels) were transformed into world pitch distances. A calibration was built on the field's reference marks acting as control points. It was calculated for each group in the classical SSG (pre-test) and in each training condition. Effect sizes (partial eta squared) and ANOVA with post-hoc test (LSD) were performed using SSPS.

Results. Table 2 presents *Ball Advance* mean ($\pm$ SD) results per group (pre-test) and per training condition. During the pre-test, *Ball Advance* did not present statistical significant effect, so that the different groups' level of coordination could be considered as equivalent. The *Ball Advance* indicator revealed a high effect size value on the training conditions factor, so that we ran follow-up analyses. The ANOVA and post-hoc analyses revealed that *Ball Advance* in SSPG was longer in C4 than in C3 ($p < .05$), than in C2 ($p < .01$), and than in C1 ($p < .01$). Surprisingly, *Ball Advance* in SSPG without 4P strategy (C2) was shorter than in C1, in the classical SSG ($p < .05$).

Table 2. Ball Advance within the field for each possession of a ball in a team (in meters).

Ball advance		M	SD	F	p	Partial η^2
Pre-test	G1	14,8	6,98	0,07	ns	0,04
	G2	15,4	6,48			
	G3	14,5	6,80			
	G4	15,4	5,35			
Training conditions	C1	16,1	6,85	11,6	.00	1,67
	C2	12,6	7,85			
	C3	17,4	5,62			
	C4	20,8	6,02			

Conclusion. First, our results suggested that coaches should carefully designed SSG, and ensure their representativeness. Because some SSPG presented high level of constraints (C2), youth players performed less than in a usual SSG (C1). Second, youth players' decisions and coordination were favoured in SSPG when the 4P strategy promoted positioning and picturing (C3 & C4). Furthermore, the results highlighted the interest of video feedbacks. Video-cued artefacts embedded in the coaching process, seems to be useful for *picturing* the relevant configuration of play (C4).

4.3   Video Feedbacks Vs Ideas Debate for Enhancing Coordination in Team?

A second study consisted in comparing the effects of an explicit or an implicit learning on collective coordination in adult players [14]. Within a SSPG, coaches provided help to the players through two types of pedagogical aids. Ideas debates were conducted aiming at promoting explicit learning; they were supposed to lead to shared knowledge. Video feedbacks were used in order to favour shared recognition of relevant configurations of play through an implicit learning.

Setting and Participants. The participants of this study consisted of 40 postgraduate students aged 20–23 years, from the "soccer special course" in the third year of the sport sciences curriculum, at the Sport Sciences Faculty in West Brittany University in France. The participants of the study were of mixed ability and had long experiences of soccer (10–14 years) before the unit commenced. They were randomly affected to two groups. An experimented teacher taught the content for each group. Both of the teachers possessed a soccer coaching certification and several years of soccer coaching experience. The second author supported the teachers with the integration of the video-based technology within the courses. The first author was present at each lesson to ensure teacher's fidelity to the design of the session.

Procedure. The two groups practiced a specific SSPG aiming at enhancing the progression of the ball within the midfield. Previous observations and performance analysis had conducted the teachers to choose and advocate the need for passing the ball through defensive line, when defenders adopted a zone defence. The course was divided into two sessions of 45 min. The SSPG was played 9 *vs* 9, and called "the *Babyfoot*" The area was a 42 × 27 meters rectangle divided into 6 areas. In the SSPG, the players are positioned within the inner zones depending on their tasks in the team (3 defenders, 3 midfielders, 2 forwards). Each team is allowed to score in any of their 2 goals, despite the goalkeeper. The "goalkeeper" did not use his hands. Moreover, two lateral players were free, outside the limits of the game, and could help each team keeping the possession of the ball within each zone. A main constraint was supposed to lead the player to identifying the relevant configuration of play related to the coach objective: the players had to pass the ball without any control if they wanted to reach the next zone. The design of this SSG and the parameters for each constraint were obtained prior to experimentation; task and contents were tested with other students from the 2nd year of the curriculum (Fig. 8).

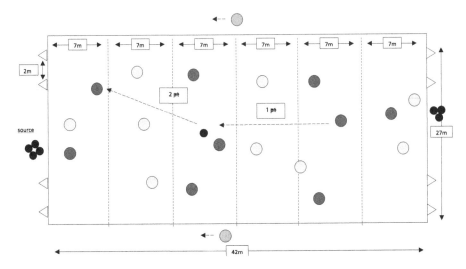

Fig. 8. The baby-foot, a small-sided positioned game.

Conditions. The two training conditions were: C1, practicing the SSPG and furnishing pedagogical aids through ideas debate; C4, practicing the SSPG and furnishing pedagogical aids though video feedbacks.

Data collection. All the games were videotaped from a fixed and high position. Video-recorded images were transferred to a digital support for notational analyses. We tracked the ball position, and noted the performance of each for each possession of a ball: 0, the defenders lost the ball; 1 point the defenders passed the ball to the midfield players; 2 points, the midfield players passed the ball to the forwards. Each time part of team recognized an opportunity to pass the ball toward the next zone and coordinated themselves, the ball reached the next zone through the defensive line. It was considered as an objective measure of collective tactical skills learning. These measures were collected during the first 20 min in the beginning of the first session (pre-test), and during 20 min at the end of the second session (post-test).

Data Analysis. Effect sizes (partial eta squared) and ANOVA were performed using SSPS on team performances for the pre-test and the post-test.

Results. During the pre-test, teams' performances did not present statistical significant effect, so that the different groups' level of coordination could be considered as equivalent. Both of the groups progress significantly. For the post-test, effect size on the training conditions factor was moderate ($\eta^2 = 0,036$). The ANOVA and post-hoc analyses suggested that video feedback provided more efficient aid than ideas debates ($F = 3,99$; $p < .05$).

Conclusion. Such a SSPG presented high level of constraints and technology support seemed to be helpful for the players. Furthermore, the results highlighted the interest of visual pedagogical aids more than verbal intervention such as ideas debate. Video

feedbacks embedded in the coaching process, seems to be useful for sharing configurations of play between teammates.

5 Conclusions

The aim of this chapter was to present some advances from NDM for tactical skills
training in team sports. Consequently, it was demonstrated that the 4P strategy and
included video feedbacks could promote an intuitive and coordinated decision-making
by highlighting configurations of play. Thus, these findings emphasized that the
Intuitive and Coordinated Decision-Making (ICDM) model (see Fig. 1) issued from
NDM is a consistent background for the 4P strategy and for tactical skills training.

Finally, four key-points have been highlighted:

(1) Whereas many frameworks in sport sciences have focused on specific factors of
    team and players performance (e.g. perceptions, knowledge, memory capabilities,
    behaviours, ...), the ICDM model described players' action as the result of a
    global, multi-determined and contextually embedded experience. For instance a
    defender in soccer use different cues such as the distance from his attackers, the
    trajectory and the ball speed, according to his own capabilities to jump, and may
    recognize the situation as familiar, not in a deliberative way, but in a "blink of an
    eye". So doing he is able to match immediately the situation and a typical action,
    connected as a typical schema in his memory. Furthermore, in many situations in
    team sports players have to share significant configurations of play to be able to
    coordinate themselves.
(2) Small-Sided Games are appropriate tools for training this kind of tactical skills.
    Nevertheless it is a challenge for coaches to design carefully appropriate SSGs.
    High level of constraints may take the SSG away from the realistic experience of
    the game, despite the fact that the attempted behaviour is provoked. Yet, limited
    evidence is available for the actual "representativeness" of SSG's for full-sized
    matches, and the notion of Small-Sided Positioned Games has been advanced to
    favour the link between the training sessions and the competitive matches.
(3) Despite coaches and teachers may use a large range of models for tactical skills
    training, it is clear that following one model or another favours different processes
    of decision-making and learning. Whereas some models favour learning by
    understanding (e.g., TGfU), or learning by adapting (e.g., LCA), our 4P strategy
    leads to learning by experiencing. The most important for tactical skills training
    seems to promote implicit learning through cumulative experiences within the
    games (i.e., *Practicing*). When they stop the games coaches' interventions should
    be concise, and visual more than verbal: just *Picturing*. Explicit learning can play
    additional roles. *Positioning* the training session consists in sense making before
    the game. At the end of the game, *post-analysing* may help players to put their
    experiences into words. Reminding and sharing experiences should lead to shared
    knowledge between teammates and between coaches and teammates, and should
    to prepare transfer of tactical skills toward other settings.

(4) The role of technological supports depends on the coaching or the teaching style. Within the 4P strategy, our findings suggested that video feedback might reinforce players' experiences. A short footage may allow action recall, viewpoints change, or display of unperceived information. Our finding suggested that such technological supports embedded in real training field help players to recognize relevant configuration of play.

Future research could also introduce other technology support within the 4P strategy. At the first step, motion analysis from previous matches, or notational analysis could be used for goal setting and positioning the training device. At the fourth step, debriefing could start with video footages: ideas debate is stimulated when ones can see his own behaviour or his teammates' performances, and sharing in promoted thanks to viewpoint changes [22].

Acknowledgements. This Synthesis Arises from Teamwork. Thanks to Coaches Y. Bourgis, L. Plassart, a. Rimasson, N. Royer, and to C. Bossard, C. Dekeukelaere, M. Le Menn, and T. Kerivel from My Lab.

References

1. Raab, M.: Thinck SMART, not hard- a review of teaching decision-making in sport from an ecological rationality perspective. Phys. Educ. Sp. Ped. **12**(1), 1–22 (2007)
2. Davids, K., Araújo, D., Correia, V., Vilar, L.: The science of team games: how small-sided games enhance acquisition of movement and decision-making skills. Ex. Sp. Sc. Rev. **41**(3), 1–8 (2013)
3. Travassos, B., Duarte, R., Vilar, L., Araujo, D., Davids, K.: Practice task design in team sports: representativeness enhanced by increasing opportunities for action. J. Sp. Sc. **30**(13), 1447–1454 (2013)
4. Grehaigne, J.-F., Godbut, P., Bouthier, D.: The teaching and learning of decision making in team sports. Quest **53**, 59–76 (2001)
5. Kermarrec, G., Roure, C.: L'entraînement et l'enseignement de la prise de décision dans les jeux sportifs collectifs. L'usage des situations de jeux réduits à l'épreuve des modèles théoriques et des résultats de la recherche en sciences du sport. eJRIEPS **37**, 58–79 (2016)
6. Renshaw, I., Araújo, D., Button, C., Chow, J.Y., Davids, K. Moy, B.: Why the constraints-led approach is not teaching games for understanding: a clarification. Phys. Ed. Sp. Ped. **20** (2015). doi:10.1080/17408989.2015.1095870
7. Klein, G.: Naturalistic decision making. Hum. Fact. **50**(3), 456–460 (2008). doi:10.1518/001872008X288385
8. Kermarrec, G., Bossard, C.: Defensive soccer players decision-making: a naturalistic study. J. Cog. Eng. Dec. Mak. **8**(2), 187–199 (2014). doi:10.1177/1555343414527968
9. Salas, E., Nichols, D.R., Driskell, J.E.: Testing three team training strategies in intact teams: a meta-analysis. Small Gr. Res. **38**, 471–488 (2007)
10. Salas, E., Diaz Granados, D., Klein, C., Burke, S., Stagl, K., Goodwin, G., Halpin, S.M.: Does team training improve team performance? a meta-analysis. Hum. Fact. **50** 903–933 (2008). doi:10.1518/001872008X37500
11. Endsley, M.R.: Toward a theory of situation awareness in dynamic systems. Hum. Fact. **37**, 32–64 (1995)

12. Macquet, A.C., Stanton, N.A.: Do the coach and athlete have the same «picture» of the situation? Distributed Situation Awareness in an elite sport context. App. Erg. **45**, 724–733 (2014)
13. De Keukelaere, C., Kermarrec, G., Bossard, C., G., Pasco, D., Loor, P.: Formes, contenus et évolution du partage au sein d'une équipe sportive de haut-niveau. [Forms, contents and dynamic of sharing within an expert team in a sport setting] Le Tr. Hum. **76,** 227–255 (2013)
14. Kermarrec, G., Kerivel, T., Bossard, C.: Apprentissage collaboratif et développement de la coordination au sein d'équipes sportives en formation universitaire, Carr. de l'E. (2017, in revision)
15. Hogarth, R.: Educating intuition, The Un. of Chicago Press (2001)
16. Kermarrec, G.: Enhancing tactical skills in soccer: advances from the naturalistic decision making approach. In: Proceedings of the 6th International Conference on Applied Human Factors and Ergonomics, Las Vegas (2015)
17. Bossard, C., Kermarrec, G., De Loor, P., Benard, R., Tisseau, J.: Sport, performance et conception de simulations participatives: illustration dans le domaine du football avec l'environnement virtuel CoPeFoot. Intellect. **2**(52), 97–117 (2009)
18. Bossard, C., Kermarrec, G., Buche, C., Tisseau, J.: Transfer of learning in virtual environments: a new challenge. Virt. Real. **2**, 151–161 (2008)
19. Fadde, P.J.: Interactive video training of perceptual decision-making in the sport of baseball. Tech. Inst. Cog. Learn. **4**, 237–256 (2006)
20. Harvey, C., Gittins, C.: Effects of Integrating Video-Based Feedback into a Teaching Games for Understanding Soccer Unit. Ag. PE Sp. **16**(3), 271–290 (2014)
21. Groom, R., Cushion, C., Nelson, L.: The delivery of video-based performance analysis by England youth soccer coaches: towards a grounded theory. J. App. Sp. Psy. **23**(1), 16–32 (2011)
22. Kermarrec, G., Bossard, C.: Shared understanding and coordination in team sports. contribution of viewpoints changes and shared information displays for team situation awareness training. In: ICSport 2014-Proc. of the 2th International Conference on Sport Sciences and Technology Support, Rome, Italy, October 26–28 (2014)
23. Kermarrec, G., Plassart, L.: Enhancing intuitive and coordinated decision-making in team sport: from the research to the field with the 4P strategy. In: ICSport 2015-Proceedings of the 3th International Conference on Sport Sciences and Technology Support, Lisbon, Portugal, 14–16 October (2015)

A Novel Approach to the Automatic Analysis of Tactics and Actions in Team Sports

D. Vallejo[1]([✉]), G. Alises[1], J.A. Albusac[2], C. Glez-Morcillo[1], and J.J. Castro-Schez[1]

[1] Faculty of Computer Science, University of Castilla-La Mancha,
Paseo de la Universidad 4, 13071 Ciudad Real, Spain
David.Vallejo@uclm.es
[2] School of Mining and Industrial Engineering, University of Castilla-La Mancha,
Plaza Manuel Meca 1, 13400 Almadén, Ciudad Real, Spain

Abstract. There can be little doubt that technology has made a contribution towards improving the preparation that professionals who have dedicated their lives to professional sports receive, both from a technical and a performance point of view. This improvement has taken place mainly on an individual level by means of tools that enable, for example, the performance of an elite sportsperson to be monitored. This monitoring process enables highly valuable information to be obtained from data collected by said tools that both the sportsperson and trainer can use for creating a process of continuous improvement. However, from the team sports viewpoint, in which success or failure depends to a large extent on coordinating efforts and using collective tactics and strategies, monitoring actions and behaviour poses a significant challenge. In light of this, an approach based on the automatic detection and analysis of situations and events in team sports has been put forward in this article. In this way, trainers of, for example, a professional football team would have a tool at their disposal which would have the potential to tell automatically if the players behaved according to the tactics and strategies set before a game. To do so, this approach has come to fruition by means of an expert system made up of a reasoning core that uses a knowledge base in which what a player should ideally do according to what has been stated by the trainer, is defined. In this knowledge base, Fuzzy Logic is defined as, a conventionality that allows the way in which human beings think to be represented and drastically bridges the gap there is between the human expert or trainer and machine. The system designed has been used in the specific domain of professional football to detect and analyse situations in which both individual players and the team as a whole are contemplated. The results obtained have allowed the way the players behave on the games field to be automatically assessed according to the knowledge previously passed on to them by the trainer.

Keywords: Team sports · Football · Event understanding · Expert systems · Fuzzy logic

© Springer International Publishing AG 2016
J. Cabri and P. Pezarat Correia (Eds.): icSPORTS 2015, CCIS 632, pp. 126–141, 2016.
DOI: 10.1007/978-3-319-52770-3_9

1   Introduction

A few years ago the huge impact that technology has in the sporting world today seems unthinkable. If, for example, a famous retired tennis player were to check firsthand how Hawk-Eye technology can answer if the ball fell inside or outside the court, he or she would have wondered, why couldn't this have been done before? Indeed, the tentacles of technology have more than infiltrated into any type of sporting event, whether it be amateur or professional. From the most basic technology, such as, for example, the use of digital scoreboards to manage the state of the game, through to highly complex technological solutions, such as those that create behaviour models for the players with the aim of improving their performance, technology is an essential support in the sporting field. From a professional point of view, this support is reflected essentially from three perspectives, which coincide with the main roles adopted in a large part of the sports there are nowadays: (i) player (ii) trainer, (iii) referee and (iv) spectator.

Professional players use technology to improve their performance or to train more effectively. For example a javelin thrower can make use of a movement analysis system to study if the throwing angle used was the optimum one or not according to other important parameters such as, for example, his or her run up speed or wind resistance. A professional billiards player can use an Augmented Reality system [1] which digitally draws the possible trajectory of the ball according to the cue direction. Moreover, all this is done before the ball is hit! Trainers benefit from automatic tools to find out the player's statistics, such as, for example, the distance covered, or the number of passes successfully made in ball sports. Furthermore, digital boards are also habitually used to explain tactics and strategies that players must follow, thereby saving time with respect to more traditional alternatives.

From the point of view of the referee, technology has enormously facilitated the assessment of game rules thereby avoiding disputes between players and conflicts that arise after seeing a replay on TV of the problematic move. The aforementioned Hawk-Eye in tennis is a highly representative example. Photofinish in athletics or the use of computerized vision techniques to detect if a player is offside (behind the defence line) when playing football (see Fig. 1) are other important examples. Finally, the spectator also benefits from technology since a highly widespread trend nowadays consists in superimposing digital information onto real sports pictures, with occasional use of Augmented Reality. For example, in sailing or American football, this approximation is used frequently.

The fruit of our labour presented in this article is a system that can be customised depending on the team sport to be analyzed. Particularly, we have deployed our system to analyze and evaluate events in the football domain. This system has been named SIDANE and focuses on the role of the football trainer. Essentially, the aim of SIDANE is to facilitate the work of these professionals via automatic analysis of situations in which the players become involved. However, SIDANE can easily be transferred to other team sports in which there are a ball to guide how the game develops.

Nowadays, professional football has developed in such a way that the concept of team has taken on, if possible, greater importance. Physical preparation of elite football players is very demanding and, although on a technical level a player may shine at specific moments, it is the team as a whole that makes the difference in championships and tournaments of a significant duration. In this way, the role of the trainer takes on special importance when facing matches and preparing both tactics and strategy for his or her players. To increase the possibility of success when facing these tasks, the trainers do not hesitate to use this new technology with the purpose of communicating their instructions to the players in the most practical and efficient way possible. From the technological support point of view, nowadays there are tools that are automatically capable of following a player at all times [6], measure the distance covered [2], jot down the number of passes made in a match [7], or even monitor the work profile of the player [4].

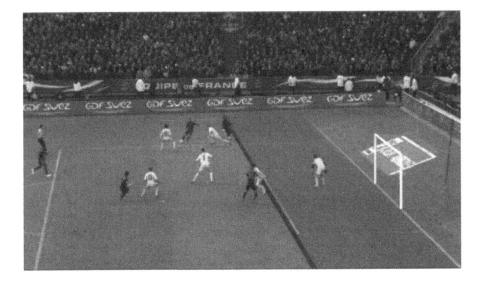

Fig. 1. Offside automatic detection.

However, it would be desirable to have higher level behaviour analysis tools, that is, those that will study when a player behaves as he or she should when faced with a certain situation, in keeping with the tactical vision and the strategy of his or her trainer. A simple example in the football world could be the goal shot. In this context, a tool that will analyse when a player should take a goal shot could analyse factors such as the distance to the goal, the number of opponent players blocking the shot or even, if there is any unmarked teammate located in a better position to take a shot at goal. Nowadays, this type of information is extracted manually by making notes on the video recording while the match took place. In this way, the trainer can justify to his or her players when they do well and when not. Unfortunately, this task, normally carried out by the trainers support team, is very tedious and prone to errors.

This is the main driving force behind SIDANE, the expert system presented in this work whose aim is to accurately analyse the actions of football players. For this purpose, at the core of SIDANE, there is a reasoning engine based on rules that determine how a player should ideally behave in given situations. The conventionality used in SIDANE is Fuzzy Logic [17], a multivalued logic that allows approximated reasoning to be carried out, using linguistic labels, instead of exact reasoning. In this way, rules can be established such as the following: if a player is surrounded by a certain number of opponent players, then he or she should pass the ball so as not to lose it. Fuzzy Logic allows the knowledge necessary for a software system to automatically analyse its input data, to be shown in a way that is very similar to how a human expert would do it. This is a highly important advantage when reducing the distance between people and machines.

The remainder of this article is structured in the following manner. In Sect. 2 there is a description of a study of related work, with special emphasis on those proposals in which there is an attempt to carry out some kind of automatic analysis in the world of football. In Sect. 3 there is a detailed discussion on what SIDANE consists of as an expert system, what is its architecture, how its reasoning engine works and what is the knowledge base that has been used as a starting point for reflecting the instructions given by the trainer. Then, in Sect. 4 the experimental results obtained when assessing SIDANE are described. The article finishes with Sect. 5, in which the conclusions arrived at are commented on and some future lines of work are presented.

2   Related Work

The state of the art as regards automatic analysis of situations in the sporting field and, specifically, in football, has made plenty of progress in recent years. In this context, it is worth stressing the importance of the tracking process as this is fundamental for locating the players and the ball at every moment [12]. This process is carried out by sophisticated Computer Vision systems which analyse the different pictures or frames that make up the video and which are captured by a multitude of cameras, which are strategically placed on the football pitch. In this context, the authors T. D'Orazio y M. Leo made a complete review of the state of the art that the reader may consult [6].

From a data obtaining point of view static cameras may be used or those used for broadcasting matches. For example, it is common enough to use fixed cameras whose fields of vision overlap, just as is discussed in [15]. However, it is perfectly possible to use the broadcasting cameras themselves, such as in [3], where the authors considered an artificial system used to analyse the 2006 World Cup matches with the purpose of positioning the players at all times. On this point, it must be emphasized that regardless of the data source, there are traditional problems that any algorithm must tackle, such as, for example the ever present occlusions or variations in the lighting sources. One work which is representative of an attempt to tackle this problem is discussed in [8], where the authors considered an algorithm made up of different steps, from a lower to higher level of abstraction, so as to, finally, obtain the position of every player on the game field.

Another large branch of activities that revolves around the tracking process is concerned with the use of hardware devices as a common denominator, which are incorporated into the player itself or the ball, instead of analysing pictures. For example, it is possible to use miniscule transmitters, such as is discussed in [13], to directly and with little scope for error, obtain the position of the players. Essentially, this approach is closely linked to GPS systems.

From an architecture perspective this layer of tracking is used as a base for other layers that have a greater level of abstraction whose aim is a higher level analysis. Then, for example, the position of the players and that of the ball could be used to *feed* an intelligent algorithm which will automatically determine in which position of the game field the player is making most effort. Another more complex example could be based on an algorithm that automatically obtains the degree of pressure from the team that does not possess the ball at each moment. Essentially, the trainer of a football team can use this knowledge to improve the preparation of tactics and strategy for his or her team, thereby saving a great deal of time as regards the traditional alternative which consists of viewing videos and making commentaries manually.

A significant amount of researchers are interested in obtaining statistical data that allows the tactical information to be used by the trainers to be extrapolated so as to improve the performance of their team. For example, in [18] the authors considered the concept of *added trajectory* to extract tactical information in situations in which a team has scored a goal. Another large field of study revolves around the analysis of the individual skills of the players. In this context, an important item is possession of the ball, since, a priori, greater possession of the ball implies greater control of the game and, therefore, greater probability of winning. To minimize the manual work derived from this task, the authors [16] put forward a semi-automatic system capable of calculating ball possession by each player from the information obtained from the television cameras. Other related work is discussed in [14], which is focused in this case on analysing the speed of the players during the game.

Beyond this individual study, the system put forward by M. Beetz et al. is worth mentioning, in which the real time video streaming analysis is considered in order to recognize activities and events [3]. This concept of *event* is especially important for the state of the art of this type of systems to make progress. With the work mentioned above, the system designed uses a reasoning engine based on first order logic to determine if a situation that was learnt previously has taken place in the match under analysis. For example, the authors comment on the examples of events the opportunity of *scoring a goal* or the situation in which a player is *under pressure*. The system maintains a series of rules that are *fired*

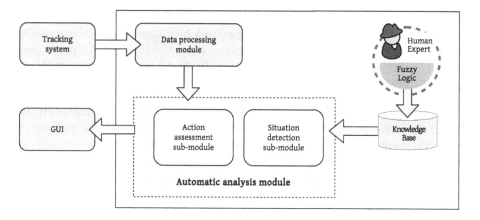

Fig. 2. Architecture overview of SIDANE.

to calculate the probability of each event handled by the situation occurring in relation to the real situation under analysis.

Other works related with the above approach are discussed in [10,11], respectively. Both work in this case with simulated data obtained from the famous competition Robocup (http://www.robocup.org), in which there are leagues both for physical robots and for virtual players which are simulated by means of sophisticated algorithms. It is worth emphasizing that in these works events such as the *average distance covered* or *possession* by each player to automatically analyse if a situation is to his or her advantage or not, are studied and detected. Another representative event, associated with automatical assessment of the *offside event*, is discussed in [5]. This work is orientated, however, to facilitating assistance to referees when assessing if there is an offside situation or not.

3   Automatic Analysis of Events

3.1   Overview

SIDANE is an expert system for the analysis and automatic assessment of situations and events in the world of football. As will be discussed further on, SIDANE is capable of, for example, detecting when a player must pass the ball and when not. For this purpose, SIDANE makes use of an expert knowledge base, defined taking into account the instructions from the football trainer, and an inference system based on rules that determine when a player is behaving well and when not. Figure 2 graphically shows the SIDANE architecture taking into account the stream of information, that is, from obtaining raw data, using for, example cameras, until high level knowledge is created such as that commented upon in the previous example.

Initially, the *tracking system* is that responsible for obtaining the position of all the players and of the ball in the games area at every moment. In other words, the responsibility this system has could consist in transforming the video streams captured by the cameras into 3D information which shows the position of the players and the ball. The tracking system is outside the scope of this paper, but the SIDANE architecture has been designed to guarantee incorporation of any tracking system. Below, the *data processing module* normalizes the information relative to said positions, in such a way that they are all found to be in the range [0.0, 0.0, 0.0] and [1.0, 1.0, 1.0]. Moreover, this sub module stores all the information received by the tracking system in a database with the purpose of making, if necessary, a forensic analysis of the data stored.

The *automatic analysis module* is the real heart of SIDANE and is made up of a reasoning system capable of detecting and analysing interesting football situations from a tactical and strategical point of view. For this purpose, and as shown in Fig. 2, this module uses a previously defined knowledge base that houses a series of rules. These rules determine if the ideal behaviour of the football player is in accordance with the criteria of his or her trainer. The mathematical conventionality that sustains both the reasoning system and the knowledge base is Fuzzy Logic [17]. Said conventionality is an extension of Boolean logic that allows dealing with uncertainty and vagueness of real world problems. For example, from a semantics point of view it is more practical to state that the ball is *close* to the goal than state that the ball is 1.34 m from it. In the following section this conventionality will be studied in greater depth.

This behaviour analysis module encompasses, in turn, two other sub modules. The first of these is the *situations detection sub-module*, responsible for detecting what is happening in the game area. For example, the reader may think of the classical offside situation. The second sub-module is the *actions assessment sub-module*, responsible for assessing if the player took the right decision in accordance with that defined by the knowledge base and within the context of the previously detected situation. For example, the reader may consider the situation in which the central defence remains back, so offside does not apply and the forward of the opponent team is enabled to act.

Finally, SIDANE provides a user graphics interface that enormously facilitates the detection of errors made by the players and that, additionally, provides detailed information of their states at every moment. It is worth emphasizing that the SIDANE architecture has been designed with special consideration for scalability maintaining a high degree of independence among the modules inserted and defining some simple interfaces that enable other modules to be incorporated.

3.2   Knowledge Base and Reasoning Engine

Fuzzy Logic [17], put forward by professor Zadeh in 1965, has been the conventionality chosen as the focal point for SIDANE. Essentially, the main feature of Fuzzy Logic is it allows the quantification of imprecise values of our language, such as *much*, *little*, or *too much*, adapting itself better to real world problems than traditional logic, which only allows for two possible values: true (1) and false (0). In this context, the human brain has a great ability to interpret and

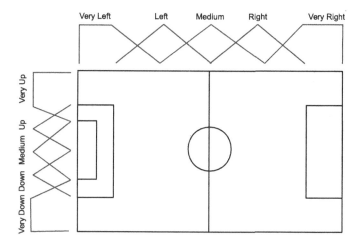

Fig. 3. Fuzzy division of the soccer field.

solve complex situations without needing to handle numerical values. It is precisely from this consideration, that the *computing with words* stream arose, to which Fuzzy Logic adapts perfectly with the concepts of *linguistic variables* and *fuzzy rules*.

In the problem dealt with in this paper, a linguistic variable could be the *attitude* of the player which, in turn, could take the values of *defensive, neutral, offensive* and *very offensive*, for example. Subsequently, this variable could be used in a fuzzy rule of the type "IF the attitude of the player is very offensive AND the distance to the goal is short, THEN, make a goal shot". This knowledge definition model is significantly close to the expert in the domain, that is, the trainer, which drastically reduces the gap between the latter and the machine. In this paper the choice of Fuzzy Logic as a knowledge representation conventionality is complemented with the inference method of Mamdani [9]. Essentially, this method is responsible for (i) changing numerical values to fuzzy values, (ii) making the reasoning process fuzzy and finally, (iii) changing the fuzzy values obtained into numerical values that can be interpreted once again by a machine.

Figure 3 shows the fuzzy division of the game area into different areas according to two independent linguistic variables: X_Pos and Y_Pos. In this way, a forward that attacks the goal on the right will normally be situated in the values *Right* or *Very Right* of the Y_Pos variable, with less likelihood of retreating to defend and that, therefore, the Y_Pos variable takes values of *Medium, Left* or *Very Left*. This type of basic variables are the first level of the knowledge base defined in this paper. The definition of another example of a basic variable denominated *Attitude*, is shown in the Fig. 4. Here, the possible values of said variable are *Defensive, Neutral* and *Offensive*.

The rules of the knowledge base of this first level are used to determine the occurrence of states or basic actions. Rules 3 and 4 of Fig. 5 show two basic examples. With rule 4, SIDANE is capable of inferring that if a player has

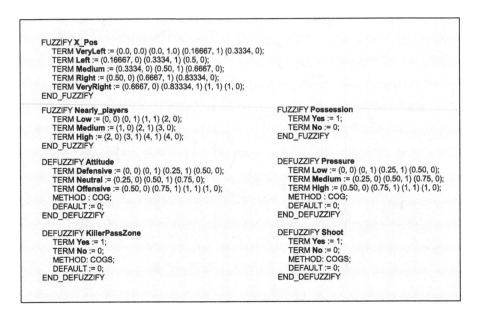

FUZZIFY X_Pos
    TERM VeryLeft := (0.0, 0.0) (0.0, 1.0) (0.16667, 1) (0.3334, 0);
    TERM Left := (0.16667, 0) (0.3334, 1) (0.5, 0);
    TERM Medium := (0.3334, 0) (0.50, 1) (0.6667, 0);
    TERM Right := (0.50, 0) (0.6667, 1) (0.83334, 0);
    TERM VeryRight := (0.6667, 0) (0.83334, 1) (1, 1) (1, 0);
END_FUZZIFY

FUZZIFY Nearly_players
    TERM Low := (0, 0) (0, 1) (1, 1) (2, 0);
    TERM Medium := (1, 0) (2, 1) (3, 0);
    TERM High := (2, 0) (3, 1) (4, 1) (4, 0);
END_FUZZIFY

FUZZIFY Possession
    TERM Yes := 1;
    TERM No := 0;
END_FUZZIFY

DEFUZZIFY Attitude
    TERM Defensive := (0, 0) (0, 1) (0.25, 1) (0.50, 0);
    TERM Neutral := (0.25, 0) (0.50, 1) (0.75, 0);
    TERM Offensive := (0.50, 0) (0.75, 1) (1, 1) (1, 0);
    METHOD : COG;
    DEFAULT := 0;
END_DEFUZZIFY

DEFUZZIFY Pressure
    TERM Low := (0, 0) (0, 1) (0.25, 1) (0.50, 0);
    TERM Medium := (0.25, 0) (0.50, 1) (0.75, 0);
    TERM High := (0.50, 0) (0.75, 1) (1, 1) (1, 0);
    METHOD : COG;
    DEFAULT := 0;
END_DEFUZZIFY

DEFUZZIFY KillerPassZone
    TERM Yes := 1;
    TERM No := 0;
    METHOD: COGS;
    DEFAULT := 0;
END_DEFUZZIFY

DEFUZZIFY Shoot
    TERM Yes := 1;
    TERM No := 0;
    METHOD: COGS;
    DEFAULT := 0;
END_DEFUZZIFY

Fig. 4. Examples of fuzzy variables in the knowledge base. The adopted notation is related to the Fuzzy Control Language (FCL).

possession of the ball and the number of opponents that are close to him or her is high, then the pressure level is high. The SIDANE knowledge base maintains more rules to determine the different pressure values according to if the number of close opponents is high or not. See how these type of rules are really simple to express for the trainer, which hugely facilitates their incorporation into the SIDANE fuzzy knowledge base.

Now pay attention to rule 10 shown equally in Fig. 5. This rule may seem more complex because the number of antecedents is greater, but in reality it is also rather simple. Rule 10, together with other similar rules included in the knowledge base, are used so that SIDANE infers when a player is found in an area of the field where it is suitable to make the so called *killer pass* and when not. This classic footballer move consists in passing the ball to a forward in such a way that the latter can score a goal just by pushing the ball. Obviously, this is a highly desirable situation. The rule in question assesses whether the one passing is lightly hugging a sideline and, moreover, is close to the rival goal. If this is the case, then the player is located in an area in which said pass is a desirable option.

The SIDANE knowledge base handles a second level or group of rules in which football concepts frequently worked on in football team training sessions are managed, such as for example *dangerous loss of ball*, *goal shot* or *long pass*. SIDANE is capable of automatically detecting when these situations take place and assessing if they were made at the right time or not. The actions associated with these concepts usually show yes or no type decisions, so defining them

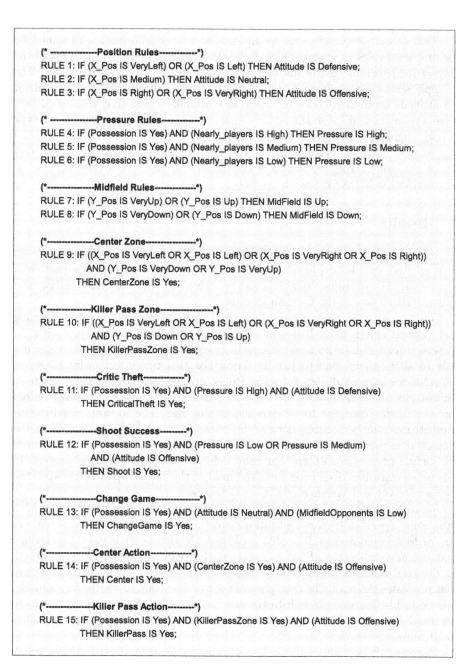

```
(* ----------------Position Rules------------*)
RULE 1: IF (X_Pos IS VeryLeft) OR (X_Pos IS Left) THEN Attitude IS Defensive;
RULE 2: IF (X_Pos IS Medium) THEN Attitude IS Neutral;
RULE 3: IF (X_Pos IS Right) OR (X_Pos IS VeryRight) THEN Attitude IS Offensive;


(* ---------------Pressure Rules------------*)
RULE 4: IF (Possession IS Yes) AND (Nearly_players IS High) THEN Pressure IS High;
RULE 5: IF (Possession IS Yes) AND (Nearly_players IS Medium) THEN Pressure IS Medium;
RULE 6: IF (Possession IS Yes) AND (Nearly_players IS Low) THEN Pressure IS Low;


(*---------------Midfield Rules------------*)
RULE 7: IF (Y_Pos IS VeryUp) OR (Y_Pos IS Up) THEN MidField IS Up;
RULE 8: IF (Y_Pos IS VeryDown) OR (Y_Pos IS Down) THEN MidField IS Down;


(*---------------Center Zone---------------*)
RULE 9: IF ((X_Pos IS VeryLeft OR X_Pos IS Left) OR (X_Pos IS VeryRight OR X_Pos IS Right))
            AND (Y_Pos IS VeryDown OR Y_Pos IS VeryUp)
        THEN CenterZone IS Yes;


(*---------------Killer Pass Zone---------------*)
RULE 10: IF ((X_Pos IS VeryLeft OR X_Pos IS Left) OR (X_Pos IS VeryRight OR X_Pos IS Right))
            AND (Y_Pos IS Down OR Y_Pos IS Up)
        THEN KillerPassZone IS Yes;


(*---------------Critic Theft------------*)
RULE 11: IF (Possession IS Yes) AND (Pressure IS High) AND (Attitude IS Defensive)
            THEN CriticalTheft IS Yes;


(*---------------Shoot Success---------*)
RULE 12: IF (Possession IS Yes) AND (Pressure IS Low OR Pressure IS Medium)
             AND (Attitude IS Offensive)
            THEN Shoot IS Yes;


(*---------------Change Game--------------*)
RULE 13: IF (Possession IS Yes) AND (Attitude IS Neutral) AND (MidfieldOpponents IS Low)
            THEN ChangeGame IS Yes;


(*---------------Center Action------------*)
RULE 14: IF (Possession IS Yes) AND (CenterZone IS Yes) AND (Attitude IS Offensive)
            THEN Center IS Yes;


(*---------------Killer Pass Action---------*)
RULE 15: IF (Possession IS Yes) AND (KillerPassZone IS Yes) AND (Attitude IS Offensive)
            THEN KillerPass IS Yes;
```

Fig. 5. Examples of fuzzy rules in the knowledge base. The adopted notation is related to the Fuzzy Control Language (FCL).

is simple. Figure 4 shows the definition of two variables associated with these actions: *killer pass* and *goal shot*. However, the most interesting part is in rule 16. This second level rule uses as an antecedent the information obtained by the first level rules (e.g. player situated in the *killer pass* area or *attitude* of the player) to determine if the player must carry out the *killer pass* or not. The example shows if the player has the ball, is in the suitable position and his or her attitude is offensive, then he or she should make a pass that will potentially leave a teammate alone so the latter can score a goal. It is precisely in this type of rule where the essence of the expert system put forward in this work can be appreciated- SIDANE is capable of assessing if the decision taken was the correct one or not, considering the action of the player and the trainer criteria which is reflected in the SIDANE knowledge base.

4   Results

As we previously stated, we designed a system that, depending on the knowledge base created, can be deployed to analyze and evaluate events in a particular team sport. For example, SIDANE was conceived to automatically analyze and evaluate situations in the football domain.

Our first aim for assessing the behaviour of SIDANE consisted in obtaining real football match data. Unfortunately, there is no public repository with the players tracking data and the research groups whom we contacted were not able to share theirs due to privacy laws. For this reason, in order to assess SIDANE we have used data from the RoboCup 2D Soccer Simulation League[1]. This league is a worldwide competition in which a range of teams of independent software agents compete to be crowned as the best. The software used in this competition allows tracking data to be obtained for all players and from the ball, so it is perfect to assess SIDANE. Likewise, the level of sophistication of the virtual players is so high that they behave as if they were real players. In this paper data has been used from the final of the RoboCup 2012 between the Helios (Japan) and WrightEagle (China) teams.

Figure 6 shows the number of detected and automatically assessed SIDANE situations. Specifically, these situations are the following: *area pass*, *dangerous loss of ball*, *killer pass* and, finally, *goal shot*. On this point it must be clarified that the *dangerous loss of ball* situation is that which triggers a counterattack by the rival team. In other words, it is a situation to be avoided by the team that possesses the ball. The *long pass* refers to a situation in which, for example, it is desirable to move the ball to the sideline opposite the game area in which, potentially, there are fewer opponent players and, therefore, more opportunities to advance.

Moreover, Figs. 7 and 9 shows two situations shown by the SIDANE graphic interface which allow what has been detected and what the players should have done to be viewed rapidly. Figure 7 shows the red player in possession of the ball and a considerable number of opponent blue players surrounding him or her.

---

[1] http://en.wikipedia.org/wiki/RoboCup 2D Soccer Simulation League.

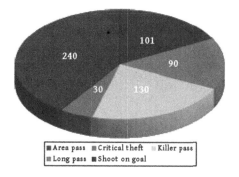

Fig. 6. Detected and assessed situations by SIDANE in the RoboCup 2012 final.

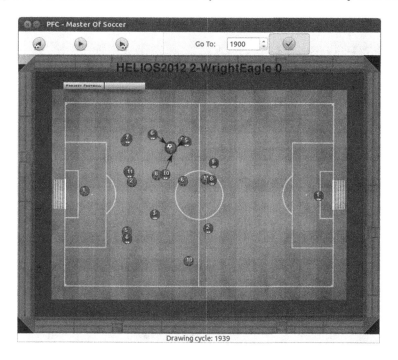

Fig. 7. Dangerous loss of ball detection (Color figure online).

In other words, SIDANE shot the rule in which there is a possibility of *dangerous loss of ball* by the other blue team. Here, the red player should pass the ball or throw it out of range of the other team to not lose it when faced with such a dangerous position. SIDANE detected and assessed 30 *dangerous loss of ball* situations in the test match. Another especially important situation from the trainer point of view is shown in Fig. 9. Here, it is desirable that the red player that has the ball makes a large run with the purpose of breathing some fresh air into the game and beginning the attack against the opponent goal. SIDANE is also capable of detecting and assessing these types of situations. In the test

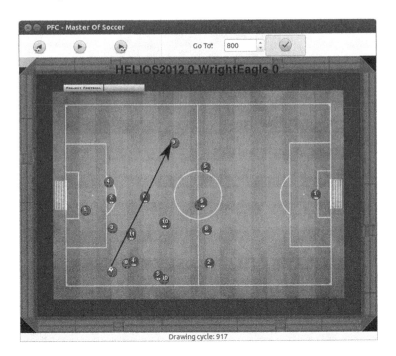

Fig. 8. Desirable long pass situation. (Color figure online)

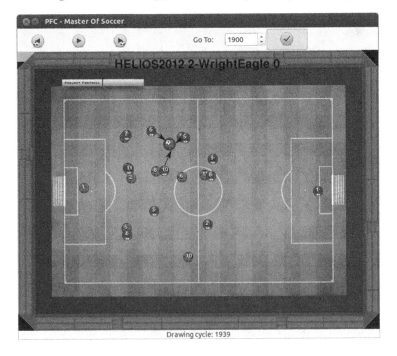

Fig. 9. Dangerous loss of ball situation. (Color figure online)

match, SIDANE detected and assessed 90 situations in which a long run was desirable (Fig. 8).

Before discussing the conclusions and the future potential lines of work associated with SIDANE the reader is advised to see a video in which situations obtained from real matches are contrasted with situations analysed by SIDANE in the RoboCup 2D Soccer Simulation League. This video is available at http://www.esi.uclm.es/www/dvallejo/sidane/video. When SIDANE detects and assesses a situation reflected in its knowledge base, the graphics interface marks the player involved with a blue circle, if the right decision is taken, or with a red circle if the wrong one is taken in accordance with that previously defined by the trainer in the knowledge base.

5   Conclusions and Future Work

In this paper an innovative approach in the automatic detection and analysis of situations and events in the field of team sports has been put forward. The main contribution made by this article is in the design and development of an expert system whose most important aim is the automatic assessment, according to knowledge previously defined by an expert or trainer, of said situations and events. This approach marks an important step forward as regards traditional techniques used to find out what is happening at each moment in a sporting event, which revolve around the moves or events being written down manually. This general objective has been reached thanks to the reasoning system incorporated into the system created in this paper, which feeds on a knowledge base that has been previously defined with Fuzzy Logic. Fuzzy Logic is a highly useful tool to show not only the knowledge of the match the expert system has, but also the inference mechanism by which new knowledge is created. To be specific, the use of if-then type rules largely enables said knowledge to be defined and bridges what at times is an unimaginable gap between the expert and machine.

The architecture of the system has been put forward with two fundamental aspects in mind: modularity and scalability. On the one hand, the modular nature of the system under discussion means the components responsible for completing the different tasks that make up the work flow can be built into the system. For example, it would be possible to incorporate a new module responsible for identifying and tracking the players being monitored. This new module could have been developed using specific Computer Vision techniques which contemplate the characteristics inherent to the sport whose events and/or actions are being monitored. In the same way, it would be possible to build a module in that, by using small hardware sensors, would know the position of the ball at all times, which is usually a fundamental issue in team sports. On the other hand, the system scalability has been contemplated from a knowledge representation point of view. In other words, the system has been designed so that the knowledge base can easily be spread with new rules associated with the analysis of new events, situations and/or behaviour. In light of this, the systems based on fuzzy rules pose a highly sound alternative for modelling and spreading the expert knowledge used to monitor said aspects.

Assessment of the system put forward in this paper has been carried out in a professional football setting. Therefore, and due to the difficulty in obtaining data for real football matches, data obtained from the RoboCup 2D Soccer Simulation League has been chosen, as data associated with tracking the players and ball is received immediately. Moreover, the level of sophistication of the algorithms used, at present, to build virtual players into this competition is so high that the football moves that occur are practically identical to those in a real match. Therefore, the analysis of a full match has enabled the system developed to be tested, working with such important concepts from a technical point of view as for example the killer pass, dangerous loss of ball, area pass or goal shot. The real potential of this system also resides in the possibility of automatically telling if a player is behaving according to knowledge passed on from the trainer, previously captured in the knowledge base using the reasoning engine designed. In other words, detection of specific situations is always complemented by their assessment, by which a comprehensive system for improving decision-taking by players in team sports has been created.

Nowadays, our effort is focused on different lines of work. In the first place, we would like to work in the field of team sports other than football. Without doubt, this would allow continuous improvement and refinement of the system created so that it can be more general and scalable. Secondly, we are especially interested in working with data from real football matches, since we think that their use would increase potential interest for these type of proposals which automatically analyse actions and behaviour. In fact, and although we are aware that the use of new prototypes may represent a real barrier for professional trainers, these type of initiatives could encourage tools to be built into the system that automate tasks that at present are carried out manually. Finally, another challenge set consists in monitoring matches in real time or confrontations between teams. Nowadays, the philosophy used is based on obtaining match data and, at a second stage, using them to analyse and assess behaviour. It would be truly interesting if this could be done straight away. To tackle this problem, a new abstraction layer would be needed which would allow computing nodes to be used, transparently, according to the system load. With this in mind, the use of ZeroC ICE, which is a communications middleware which greatly facilities the design, settings and use of distributed systems, is under consideration.

Acknowledgements. The authors would like to thank the University of Castilla-La Mancha, for funding this work under the research project GI20153014.

References

1. Azuma, R., Baillot, Y., Behringer, R., Feiner, S., Julier, S., MacIntyre, B.: Recent advances in augmented reality. IEEE Comput. Graph. Appl. **21**(6), 34–47 (2001)
2. Barros, R., Misuta, M.S., Menezes, R.P., Figueroa, P.J., Moura, F.A., Cunha, S.A., Anido, R., Leite, N.J.: Analysis of the distances covered by first division Brazilian soccer players obtained with an automatic tracking method. J. Sports Sci. Med. **6**(2), 233–242 (2007)

3. Beetz, M., Kirchlechner, B., Lames, M.: Computerized real-time analysis of football games. IEEE Perv. Comput. **4**(3), 33–39 (2005)
4. Carling, C., Bloomfield, J., Nelsen, L., Reilly, T.: The role of motion analysis in elite soccer. Sports Med. **38**(10), 839–862 (2008). Springer
5. D'Orazio, T., Leo, M., Spagnolo, P., Mazzeo, P.L., Mosca, N., Nitti, M., Distante, A.: An investigation into the feasibility of real-time soccer offside detection from a multiple camera system. IEEE Trans. Circ. Syst. Video Technol. **19**(12), 1804–1818 (2009)
6. D'Orazio, T., Leo, M.: A review of vision-based systems for soccer video analysis. Pattern Recogn. **43**(8), 2911–2926 (2010). Elsevier
7. Hughes, M., Franks, I.: Analysis of passing sequences, shots and goals in soccer. J. Sports Sci. **23**(5), 509–514 (2005). Taylor & Francis
8. Khatoonabadi, S.H., Rahmati, M.: Automatic soccer players tracking in goal scenes by camera motion elimination. Image Vis. Comput. **27**(4), 469–479 (2009). Elsevier
9. Mamdani, E.H.: Application of fuzzy algorithms for control of simple dynamic plant. Proc. Inst. Electr. Eng. **121**(12), 1585–1588 (1974)
10. Miene, A., Visser, U., Herzog, O.: Recognition and prediction of motion situations based on a qualitative motion description. In: Polani, D., Browning, B., Bonarini, A., Yoshida, K. (eds.) RoboCup 2003. LNCS, vol. 3020, pp. 77–88. Springer, Heidelberg (2004). doi:10.1007/978-3-540-25940-4_7
11. Nair, R., Tambe, M., Marsella, S., Raines, T.: Automated assistants for analyzing team behaviors. Auton. Agents Multi-agent Syst. **8**(1), 69–111 (2004). Springer
12. Prince, S.J.D.: Computer Vision: Models Learning and Inference. Cambridge University Press, Cambridge (2012)
13. Rohmer, G., Dünkler, R., Köhler, S., von der Grün, T.: A microwave based tracking system for soccer. In: Proceedings of the 18th International Technical Meeting of the Satellite Division of the Institute of Navigation (ION GNSS), pp. 2207–2212 (2001)
14. Tsai, P.S., Meijome, T., Austin, P.G.: Scout: a game speed analysis and tracking system. Mach. Vis. Appl. **18**(5), 289–299 (2007). Springer
15. Xu, M., Orwell, J., Lowey, L., Thirde, D.: Architecture and algorithms for tracking football players with multiple cameras. IEE Proc. Vis. Image Signal Process. **152**(2), 232–241 (2005)
16. Yu, X., Hay, T.S., Yan, X., Chang, E.: A player-possession acquisition system for broadcast soccer video. In: IEEE International Conference on Multimedia and Expo (ICME), pp. 522–525 (2005)
17. Zadeh, L.A.: Fuzzy logic = computing with words. IEEE Trans. Fuzzy Syst. **4**(2), 103–111 (1996)
18. Zhu, G., Huang, Q., Xu, C., Rui, Y., Jiang, S., Gao, W., Yao, H.: Trajectory based event tactics analysis in broadcast sports video. In: Proceedings of the 15th International Conference on Multimedia, pp. 58–67 (2007)

Author Index

Printed in the United States
By Bookmasters